Welfare, Exclusion and Political Agency

As a result of research and reflection on practice in social welfare and in education outside school, *Welfare, Exclusion and Political Agency* explores the connections between professional practice and wider patterns of division, exclusion and resistance.

The chapters discuss such issues as: working-class children, competence and citizenship, 1850–1914; colonization of the poor; the role of welfare in the internal control of immigration; social work and social exclusion; the experience of women practitioners in health, welfare and education; alienation and the dilemmas for formal and informal educators, and how lesbians negotiate and experience coming out.

Welfare, Exclusion and Political Agency will be essential reading for health and welfare professionals, academics and students of social work and social policy.

Janet Batsleer is a Senior Lecturer in Applied Community Studies and Women's Studies at Manchester Metropolitan University. **Beth Humphries** is a Principal Lecturer at Manchester Metropolitan University and Director of Postgraduate Studies in the Department of Applied Community Studies

The State of Welfare
Edited by Mary Langan

Nearly half a century after its post-war consolidation, the British welfare state is once again at the centre of political controversy. After a decade in which the role of the state in the provision of welfare was steadily reduced in favour of the private, voluntary and informal sectors, with relatively little public debate or resistance, the further extension of the new mixed economy of welfare in the spheres of health and education became a major political issue in the early 1990s. At the same time the impact of deepening recession has begun to expose some of the deficiencies of market forces in areas such as housing and income maintenance, where their role had expanded dramatically during the 1980s. *The State of Welfare* provides a forum for continuing the debate about the services we need in the 1990s.

Titles of related interest also in *The State of Welfare* series:

Taking Child Abuse Seriously
The Violence Against Children
Study Group

Women, Oppression and Social Work
Edited by Mary Langan and Lesley Day

Managing Poverty
The Limits of Social Assistance
Carol Walker

Towards a Post-Fordist Welfare State?
Roger Burrows and Brian Loader

Working with Men
Feminism and Social Work
Edited by Kate Cavanagh and Viviene E. Cree

Social Theory, Social Change and Social Work
Edited by Nigel Parton

Working for Equality in Health
Edited by Paul Bywaters and Eileen McLeod

Social Action for Children and Families
Edited by Crescy Cannan and Chris Warren

Child Protection and Family Support
Nigel Parton

Social Work and Child Abuse
David Merrick

Towards a Classless Society?
Edited by Helen Jones

Poverty, Welfare and the Disciplinary State
Chris Jones and Tony Novak

Welfare, Exclusion and Political Agency

Edited by Janet Batsleer and Beth Humphries

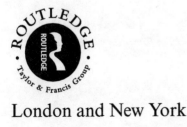

London and New York

First published 2000 by Routledge
11 New Fetter Lane, London EC4P 4EE

Simultaneously published in the USA and Canada by Routledge
29 West 35th Street, New York, NY 10001

Routledge is an imprint of the Taylor & Francis Group

© 2000 Janet Batsleer and Beth Humphries, selection and editorial
matter; individual chapters, the contributors

Typeset in Times by Taylor & Francis Books Ltd

Printed and bound in Great Britain by MPG Books Ltd, Bodmin

British Library Cataloguing in Publication Data
A catalogue record for this book is available from the British Library

Library of Congress Cataloging in Publication Data
A catalog record for this book has been requested

ISBN 0–415–19513–6 (hbk)
ISBN 0–415–19514–4 (pbk)

Contents

vi *Contents*

Contributors

Gill Aitken works as a clinical psychologist in a regional secure unit at Mental Health Services of Salford. She has an ongoing commitment to reflect on personal, professional and institutional assumptions and practices in order to develop more appropriate, less oppressive service provision. She is actively involved in various networks, lecturing and writing as part of this process.

Janet Batsleer is a senior lecturer in Applied Community Studies and Women's Studies at Manchester Metropolitan University. She is currently chair of FortySecond Street, a Manchester resource for young people experiencing mental health difficulties, which has a long tradition of participatory and innovatory practice. She is the author of *Working with Girls and Young Women in Community Settings* (Arena 1996), her attempt to prevent some recent feminist politics and activism from disappearing from the written record.

Tom Cockburn is currently a lecturer in the Department of Applied Community Studies at Manchester Metropolitan University. In 1992 he completed an MPhil (University of Manchester) on children's relationship to citizenship. In 1996 he was awarded a PhD (University of Manchester) which was an analysis of children in Manchester from the late nineteenth to early twentieth centuries. From 1996–98 he worked on a research project with young people in the Moss Side district of Manchester. His research interests are with past and present representations of children and young people, research methods and social theory.

Daryl S. Crosskill is an independent trainer specializing in working with diversity, group dynamics and identity formation. He is currently completing a PhD thesis at Manchester Metropolitan University which argues that ideas associated with colonialism are relevant to the deconstruction of ideologies underpinning the welfare state.

Debra Hayes completed a master's degree in social work and was in the probation service for seven years, before taking up a senior lecturer post at Manchester Metropolitan University in 1991. She has collaborated extensively with Greater Manchester Immigration Unit over a number of years. She has jointly organized three conferences on prisoners and deportation, on children, social work and immigration, and on health and immigration controls. Her PhD research is on Race, Health and Immigration Control and she has a number of publications in this area. Debra is joint author with Steve Cohen of *They Make You Sick: essays on immigration control and health* (MMU/GHIAU 1998).

Beth Humphries is a principal lecturer at Manchester Metropolitan University and director of postgraduate studies in the Department of Applied Community Studies. She has published in the areas of research methods and in 'empowerment' in social work. Her most recent book is *Research in an Unequal World* (1999, edited with Carole Truman and Donna M. Mertens)

Mary Issitt is a senior lecturer in the Department of Humanities and Applied Social Studies at Manchester Metropolitan University. She is currently course leader in the MA/Postgraduate Diploma in Health Promoting Practice. She worked as a practitioner in a wide range of human service contexts prior to coming into higher education. She has been conducting research and publishing in the spheres of competence and reflective practice for several years.

Steve Morgan is a senior lecturer in social work and applied community studies at Manchester Metropolitan University. He worked for ten years as a probation officer and his research background is in penology and criminal justice policy. His current work on prison autobiography has its roots in concern for the recognition of offenders as credible voices in debates about crime and offending.

Carol Packham is a teacher and youth and community worker. She is senior lecturer and route leader in youth and community work at Manchester Metropolitan University. Her specialisms are informal education, youth work involvement with schools, and participatory methodologies in community auditing. She was a member of Manchester Free School and Chair of Governors at her local primary school in Whalley Range, Manchester, where she is a voluntary youth and community worker and chair of the Community Forum.

Helen Spandler is a research student at the Discourse Unit in the Department of Psychology and Speech Pathology at Manchester Metropolitan University. She has researched and written on young people and self-harm and the mental health user movement. She has been active in socialist and mental health politics for over ten years.

Vic Tuck is a staff development officer with Solihull Social Services Department where he organizes child protection training. He has researched links between social deprivation and harm to children.

Helen Williamson is a social work practitioner working for an inner-city community drugs team in Manchester. She moved to Manchester in 1978 to undertake a BA honours degree in social science. She recently completed a master's dissertation in social work at Manchester Metropolitan University. Her research topic was experiences of lesbians of 'coming out'. Before qualifying as a social worker, Helen did a variety of work for Women's Aid and a local HIV organization. She has a keen interest in gender and sexuality issues and in raising their profile in social work.

Series editor's preface

State welfare policies reflect changing perceptions of key sources of social instability. In the first half of the twentieth century – from Bismarck to Beveridge – the welfare state emerged as a set of policies and institutions which were – in the main – a response to the 'problem of labour', the threat of class conflict. The major objective was to contain and integrate the labour movement. In the post-war decades, as this threat receded, the welfare state became consolidated as a major employer and provider of a wide range of services and benefits to every section of society. Indeed, it increasingly became the focus of blame for economic decline and was condemned for its inefficiency and ineffectiveness.

Since the end of the Cold War, the major fear of capitalist societies is no longer class conflict, but the socially disintegrative consequences of the system itself. Increasing fears and anxieties about social insta-bility – including unemployment and homelessness, delinquency, drug abuse and crime, divorce, single parenthood and child abuse – reflect deep-seated apprehensions about the future of modern society.

The role of state social policy in the Clinton–Blair era is to restrain and regulate the destructive effects of market forces, symbolized by the Reagan–Thatcher years. On both sides of the Atlantic, governments have rejected the old polarities of left and right, the goals of both comprehensive state intervention and rampant free-market individu-alism. In its pursuit of a 'third way' the New Labour government, which came to power in Britain in May 1997, has sought to define a new role for government at a time when politics has largely retreated from its traditional concerns about the nature and direction of society.

What are the values of the third way? According to Tony Blair, the people of middle England 'distrust heavy ideology', but want 'security and stability'; they 'want to refashion the bonds of community life' and, 'although they believe in the market economy, they do not believe that the only values that matter are those of the market place' (*The Times*, 25 July 1998). The values of the third way reflect and shape a traditional and conservative response to the dynamic and unpredictable world of the late 1990s.

The view expressed by Michael Jacobs, a leading participant in the revived Fabian Society, that 'we live in a strongly individualized society which is falling apart' is widely shared (*The Third Way*, London: The Fabian Society, 1998). For him, 'the fundamental principle' of the third way is 'to balance the autonomous demands of the individual with the need for social cohesion or "community"'. A key New Labour concept that follows from this preoccupation with community is that of 'social exclusion'. Proclaimed the government's 'most important innovation' when it was announced in August 1997, the 'social exclusion unit' is at the heart of New Labour's flagship social policy initiative – the 'welfare to work' programme. The preoccupation with 'social exclusion' indicates a concern about tendencies towards fragmentation in society and a self-conscious commitment to policies which seek to integrate atomized individuals and thus to enhance social cohesion.

The popularity of the concept of social exclusion reflects a striking tendency to aggregate diverse issues so as to imply a common origin. The concept of social exclusion legitimizes the moralizing dynamic of New Labour. Initiatives such as 'welfare to work', targeting the young unemployed and single mothers, emphasize individual responsibility. Duties – to work, to save, to adopt a healthy lifestyle, to do homework, to 'parent' in the approved manner – are the common themes of New Labour social policy; obligations take precedence over rights.

Though the concept of social exclusion targets a smaller section of society than earlier categories such as 'the poor' or 'the underclass', it does so in a way which does imply a societal responsibility for the problems of fragmentation, as well as indicating a concern to draw people back – from truancy, sleeping rough, delinquency and drugs, etc. – into the mainstream of society. Yet New Labour's sympathy for the excluded only extends as far as the provision of voluntary work and training schemes, parenting classes and drug rehabilitation programmes. The socially excluded are no longer allowed to be the passive recipients of benefits; they are obliged to participate in their moral reintegration. Those who refuse to subject themselves to these apparently benign forms of regulation may soon find themselves the target of more coercive interventions.

There is a further dimension to the third way. The very novelty of New Labour initiatives necessitates the appointment of new personnel and the creation of new institutions to overcome the inertia of the established structures of central and local government. To emphasize the importance of its drugs policy, the government has created the new office of Drugs Commissioner – 'Tsar' – and prefers to implement the policy through a plethora of voluntary organizations, rather than through traditional channels. Health action zones, education action zones and employment action zones are the chosen vehicles for policy innovation in their respective areas. At higher levels of government, semi-detached special policy units, think tanks and quangos play an increasingly important role.

The State of Welfare series aims to provide a critical assessment of social policy in the new millennium. We will consider the new and emerging 'third way' welfare policies and practices and the way these are shaped by wider social and economic changes. Globalization, the emergence of post-industrial society, the transformation of work, demographic shifts and changes in gender roles and family structures all have major consequences for patterns of welfare provision.

Social policy will also be affected by the demands of social movements – women, minority ethnic groups, disabled people – as well as groups concerned with sexuality or the environment. *The State of Welfare* series will examine these influences when analysing welfare practices in the first decade of the new millennium.

Mary Langan
February 1999

Acknowledgements

Much of the work for this collection of essays has been undertaken in the context of the Social Divisions Research Group, based in the Department of Applied Community Studies at Manchester Metropolitan University. We thank both those colleagues in the Group who helped with the process of thinking about issues of inequality and resistance, and the Department for allowing us and other colleagues the space to develop our understandings.

Jackie Batstone, our senior department administrator, has, on a number of occasions and again for this volume, carried out the collating, typesetting and other jobs to bring the work up to the publisher's technical standards. We very much appreciate her contribution to this collection, and are sad that it coincides with her departure from the university.

We have been sustained by a number of networks as the book has proceeded. Janet would like to thank colleagues and friends in the Women's Studies Centre at Manchester Metropolitan University; also colleagues at FortySecond Street in Manchester for the opportunities they give for new insights into the ways debates in practice change and stay the same; and Margaret Beetham for keeping her at it. Beth wishes to thank Marion for her daily support and interest in Beth's work.

We are grateful to Sony Music Publishing for kind permission to reproduce an extract from the song *4st 7lb* by the Manic Street Preachers (words by James Bradfield, Richard Edwards, Nicholas Jones and Sean Moore). The quote from *Peter Pan* is reproduced by permission of Great Ormond Street Hospital for Children.

1 Welfare, exclusion and political agency

Janet Batsleer and Beth Humphries

Introduction

This collection of essays arises from research and reflection on practice in social welfare and in education outside school, and from a desire on the part of all the contributors to explore the connections between professional practice and wider patterns of division, exclusion and resistance in modern Britain. The theoretical frameworks which framed an earlier generation's reflections on 'radical social work' or 'liberatory education' have been under pressure, and so we have been involved in a theoretical and practical project which has entailed an engagement with emerging theoretical frameworks and with accounts of 'good practice' in the field of welfare. In a situation of increasing inequality and changing professional roles, where accustomed ways of making sense of these changes have been profoundly challenged, the contributors offer their understandings of the implications, and the potential for progressive practice.

In this introduction, we set out our understanding of these material and theoretical changes, and we investigate a cluster of concepts which inform the chapters which follow. Thus we hope to contribute to a re-definition of professional roles in welfare practice – what we refer to as *critical professionals* – and to ways in which they may contribute to 'voice' and agency of those increasingly excluded from the full benefits of citizenship.

The chapter sets out discourses about welfare, welfare recipients and welfare professionals, then examines contemporary theoretical understandings. In particular it looks at the potential of Foucault's ideas for understanding contemporary society and for identifying spaces where new voices may be heard. It goes on to offer some pointers towards a role for 'critical professionals', and ends by intro-ducing the chapters which follow.

2 Janet Batsleer and Beth Humphries

Welfare, citizenship and exclusion

The evidence for deepening poverty both in Britain and across the world is irrefutable. Townsend (1993), Graham (1993), Doyal (1995), Oppenheim and Harper (1996), Leonard (1997), among others, have identified the economic, social and cultural factors which prevent people from meeting their material and psychological needs. Some of the factors limit the potential of both sexes: 'global inequalities in income and wealth, for example, as well as environmental degradation and the barriers of "race" and class that continue to divide both rich and poor countries' (Doyal 1995: 231). Others are gender specific and are apparent in a range of dimensions including paid and unpaid labour; hazards at work; violence in the home; medicine and power over women (Anthias and Yuval Davis 1992; Dalla Costa and Dalla Costa 1993; Walby 1997). At the same time, there has been a restructuring of welfare, resulting from the need to subordinate social policy to the needs of the economy and with it a shift in the constructed images and identities of recipients of welfare.

The framework of citizenship as a basis for the analysis of welfare as a development of social rights is usually associated with the work of T.H. Marshall (Marshall 1950). From another perspective, 'dependence on welfare' is a failure of citizenship, because it points to a failure of that central activity and duty of the citizen: participation in the labour market (Mead 1986; Novak 1987).

Liberal traditions of citizenship concerned with developing definitions of rights jostle with civic republican traditions of citizenship concerned with active participation in reaching the goals of a society, frequently conceived as participation in the creation of wealth through participation in the labour market. In this account, paid work is no mere economic necessity: it is also the practice of civic virtue. To be a citizen is to be included. Who then is to be included?

The discourses of welfare mark social division, inclusion and exclusion: mark 'them' and 'us' in changing and shifting ways. From the essays in this collection, it will be clear that discourses of 'professional' and 'user', of 'competent' and 'incompetent', continue to be significant. Linked to these are concepts of normality and otherness, including criminality, madness and alienness, which mark the social divisions and social sites at which borders of inclusion and exclusion can be drawn.

Discussion of 'exclusion', and to a lesser extent 'inclusion', shapes much discourse surrounding welfare, health and education currently. It is useful to acknowledge the lineage of the term 'exclusion' in welfare discourse, which terms it has displaced, and what debates and dialogues it may enable to emerge. The term 'exclusion' follows in a lineage which includes 'deprivation' and 'marginality'. It disguises and yet cannot be completely separated from discourses which reference social and political injustice more directly, such as discourses about discrimination and disadvantage. Following the rediscovery of charity as a major welfare practice, and the mobilization of self-interest through the National Lottery alongside the committed withdrawal of the state as the central welfare provider and the development of the quasi-market as a system for the provision of services, there has been a rediscovery of fear of 'the mob', the outcasts, those who have no stake in existing social relations. From a situation in which issues of welfare were legitimately understood as the concern of the whole society and of the majority of its citizens – since everyone could be understood as vulnerable to sickness, neglect, old age, unemployment – welfare services are now 'targeted' at specific groups. Interdependence is not understood as a necessary condition for autonomy and citizenship. Instead, 'dependence on welfare' – another term for social exclusion – is not a state we can all expect to enter at some point in our lives, but a position to be avoided at all costs.

Anyone who fails to escape dependence on welfare is likely to be seen as deficient in some way, some kind of failure. From the connection with the discourse of deprivation, we can hear the continuation of victim-blaming into discourses of exclusion: 'Deprived children, whether in their own homes or out of them, are the sources of social infection as real and as serious as are carriers of diphtheria and typhoid' (Bowlby, cited in Pascall 1997: 77).

The excluded ones, the outcasts – the criminals, the paedophiles, the 'care in the community cases', the lone parents on council estates, the illegal immigrants, the teenage mothers – are sometimes understood as threatening, as capable of wielding a destructive, though often passive, power which – perhaps by 'draining resources' – could undermine social coherence. So although analyses of social exclusion draw most directly on a Durkheimean model of social integration rather than on models of democracy or models which highlight social conflict over resources and power (Levitas 1996), they are shadowed and haunted by the question of power, often in the form of the creation of division and difference, of the 'other' who haunts the 'norm'. And, of course, those who are excluded can indeed threaten, with the force of abjection, of the abject created at the boundary of exclusion and inclusion (Sibley 1995). Those who are called monstrous can behave monstrously.

At the same time, those who are outside/excluded/other can draw on the humanist claims of liberal democracies to offer equality of status and fair treatment to citizens. They can speak the language of human rights and of the need to resist discrimination. They can even participate in the definition of 'need' and the debate about allocation of resources.

In Britain, one of the flagships of the New Labour government is the 'Social Exclusion Unit'. Its initial brief has been to address issues of truancy from school, the problem of rough sleepers and the problems facing the most deprived estates. 'Exclusion' is not understood as a dynamic process, or even as a category of analysis, but as a property of particular populations and areas. The antidote to exclusion, furthermore, is to be found in the operation of the labour market. To be included is to be incorporated into the system, to be found a place in the paid labour market, however flexible or marginal that place may be. Or it means to be found a place in the education system, with access to qualifications seen as the best precondition of access to the labour market. For young people aged 16–25, for lone parents with children over 5 years of age, there is to be 'no other option'. The 'gateway' to social inclusion is the 'gateway' to the labour market. 'Dependence on welfare' – that feminized sign of subordination – needs to be replaced by citizenship and participation, specifically participation in the waged labour market. Much welfare practice will be concerned with enabling the transition from welfare to work.

If the place of the citizen is in the labour market, then the space occupied by those who are excluded can be defined as not occupied by citizens. Rather, it can perhaps be understood as occupied by the 'denizens' of an underclass (Hammar 1990), who need to be confined. For those who remain undisciplined by the exigencies of the labour market, there is certainly control of the space they may occupy. This control includes hostels for rough sleepers, foyer projects for the young 'homeless and jobless' in which accommodation and training are linked, curfews for young offenders, court orders for the parents of school truants, prisons, of course, for those convicted of criminal offences and for those on remand awaiting trial, detention centres for asylum seekers and compulsory treatment in the community for the mentally ill. Britain has one of the highest prison populations in Europe (Muncie and Sparks 1991), and just as welfare policy is being modelled on the American workfare system, so the pattern of racialization of the prison population so evident in the United States can be found here. Exclusion involves the drawing of borders. Those who have been excluded/have excluded themselves, will need to be controlled. It is here that the practices of control and care are so neatly intertwined, and it is here, therefore, that the work of professionals may make the most difference. Many chapters in this collection show the operation and histories of discourses of professionalism and competence as discourses of exclusion – exclusion from school, exclusion from free society, exclusion from citizenship, exclusion from definitions of the 'normal'. In forcing division, assessing and excluding practices may well become sites not only of anger and conflict, but also of interpersonal and collective violence. They may also become sites of resistance.

Welfare and the analysis of need

Welfare systems have been analysed in relation to the settlement they enact between the market and the state as providers for human need. In this perspective, welfare is the practice of defining which human needs are to be met by a particular state and which are to be left to the mercies and neglects of the market economy (Esping-Andersen 1996). The place of welfare in ensuring the sustainability of market economies continues to be debated and analysed. Much policy in this area centres on the need to control the welfare budget, to keep it in check (rather as the unruly recipients of welfare must be kept in check), so that it does not inhibit the free development of labour markets, or inhibit free citizens and consumers with too heavy a burden of taxation. At the same time, social democratic traditions affirm the importance of health care and education to all citizens. The practice of 'needs assessment' is familiar everyday practice for many professionals in this area, and can be understood as a means of rationing resources. Juridical, administrative and technical discourses of need dominate welfare practice.

However, these discourses are changing as the practice of welfare has been restructured. Clarke (1996) has identified four important elements of this re-structuring: marketization; the development of mixed economies of welfare; the shift from formal to informal provision, including the increasing familialization of welfare; and managerialization. He argues that older definitions of professionalism have been transformed in this process: 'neither markets nor mixed economies run themselves: they require agents to make them work. In the contemporary public sector the preferred form of that agency is management. More particularly it is management as opposed to administrative bureaucracy or professionalism' (Clarke 1996: 46).

This complex process of restructuring has had implications for the role and identity of welfare professionals, and for the notion of the rational application of professional expertise to the solution of social problems. Not only did welfare professionals become increasingly despondent at the deepening poverty of their 'clients', but they have entered a regime in which they have been put on the defensive by 'the assertion of customer-centred models of provision, the fragmentations of professional tasks and the expectation that professionals can be disciplined by the creation of devolved managerial systems and new responsibilities for resource control' (Clarke 1996: 53). Moreover, professionals are perceived as needing new skills, so their education has become increasingly state regulated, to achieve 'fitness for the task', in the case of social work to an unprecedented degree. As Jones (1996) points out:

> There has been an on-going process of theoretical stripping out of the social work curriculum. In its place students are increasingly confronted with a mish-mash of methods, skills and values teaching, often lacking any coherence. Values in particular have come to occupy a strangely central position, with CCETSW appearing to believe that they can be a substitute for knowledge and understanding. There is no comparable system for social work education in the world which is nationally uniform, uninspired and tailored so closely to the requirements of major state employers.
>
> (Jones 1996: 190)

There has been a purging of 'dangerous' theories in the quest for loyalty and managerialist efficiency. Instead, a 'competence culture' dominates education in the welfare, health and education arenas (see Edwards and Usher 1994; Humphries 1997). The competency movement signals a decisive shift of power over education and training in favour of employers, business interests and the central state acting as the agent of international capital (Alexander and Martin 1995). The emphasis has moved away from critical analysis of the social and political construction of knowledge towards prescription and imposition of a narrowly defined curriculum based on approved pre-selections of knowledge and 'skills'. This, among other factors, has contributed to a general state of demoralization and exhaustion among professionals which has taken its toll in terms of undermining resistance and activism (Jones and Novak 1993).

However, there are those who are determined that their practice should continue to be informed by critical currents. Many feminist writers and, in particular, a number of black writers have continued to draw on discourses of professionalism in order to develop their own perspectives on a radical practice, distinct from both the older Fabian accounts and new market-based 'care manager' perspectives. In her important essay 'Women, welfare and the politics of need interpretation', Nancy Fraser suggests that welfare is a site which signifies the failure of the binary systems which are the basis of liberal understandings of society (public/private; state/market), and will not do as conceptualizations (Fraser 1989). Fraser writes:

> the social is a sphere of discourse about people's needs, specifically about those needs which have broken out of the domestic and/or official economic spheres that earlier contained them as 'private matters'. Thus the social is the site of discourse about problematical needs, needs which have come to exceed the apparently (but not really) self-regulating domestic and economic institutions of male dominated capitalist society.
>
> (Fraser 1989: 116)

It is this sphere – as part of the landscape of civil society – in which social workers, educators, psychologists and health workers intervene.

While it is clear that the market economy globally fails to meet basic needs and distributes this failure through certain familiar axes of inequality, the practice of welfare as 'needs assessment' can be seen as a key mechanism through which these inequalities are perpetuated. However, the essays in this volume are written at some distance from a functionalist account of welfare as simply maintaining the market economy. Welfare practice, including the definition of need, is a discursive practice in which a struggle over the distribution of resources occurs. Dominant juridical technical and administrative discourses of need are 'expert knowledges', monological discourses which separate professional from client and ensure the continuance of existing power relations of all kinds. But they are challenged by the needs discourses associated with oppositional movements, including movements of users and clients, as well as by the discourses of constituencies dedicated to reprivatizing need: strengthening the discourse of the family, for example. Critical professionals have an essential role in refusing to engage in monological discourses and 'expert' roles. In an analysis of discursive practices which leans hard on a Foucauldian account of power, the politics of needs interpretation is also a politics of discipline, control and subjectification, and always necessarily a politics of resistance.

The challenge to universal theories of oppression and resistance

Alongside these profound changes in the definition of welfare and welfare subjects and the undermining of state provision, traditional ways of theorizing social phenomena have also come under attack. The challenge to universal theories of inequality, oppression and resistance, for example, has come from two rather different and yet often allied sources. First, there is the critique of universalist perspectives associated with the critique of ethnocentric and imperialist influences on theory. For instance, feminist theorizing which proposed and analysed a universal oppression of women, as a basis for a global movement for liberation, has been subject to a swelling critique by black and Third World feminists (e.g. Amos and Parmar 1984; Carby 1982; Lorde 1984; hooks 1982; Mohanty 1991). The problem was that dominant feminist theories did not take account of difference among women, and tended to represent and analyse the experience of white Western heterosexual middle-class women as common to all women. Feminist writers have taken up these criticisms in social policy and social welfare (e.g. Carabine 1996; Dominelli 1991; Doyal 1995; Graham 1993; Lewis 1996; Price 1996; Williams 1989, 1996). From one perspective, the theorization of difference will lead to a more adequate global, universal understanding of the position of women, and the critique of false universalisms does not lead to an abandonment of the search for universal knowledges. From another position, the knowledge which matters must always be particular and located, refusing to uncover a truth about 'woman' but producing knowledges which are historically and geographically situated (Harding 1991). The implications of this critique of universal theories of oppression – for example within the family – are of major importance for practitioners, as it means the refusal of guidelines to be applied in every situation and an attentive analysis of the specific dynamics of power in each setting.

The second source of critique of universal theories of oppression and resistance can be found in postmodernism and poststructuralism. Modernist and structuralist understandings are the subject of critique because, it is claimed, they rest on an understanding of the realm of the social as a single whole about which the truth can be uncovered, and on a view of history in which change occurs through the workings out of a dialectic of progress, in which the true nature of the human becomes progressively clearer to us. The veils of illusion are discarded and our true nature becomes more plain.

The critique of this European Enlightenment model is widespread and complex, and one of the forms it has taken, which has much bearing on the practice of welfare, is the critique of essentialism. Lyotard (1979) defines postmodernism as incredulity towards meta-narratives. He argues (in many ways following Blake, Swift and other anti-modernist Enlightenment figures) that grand narratives of progress and human perfectability are no longer tenable, since they render invisible difference, opposition and plurality. Modernity has meant in practice a Eurocentric, patriarchal and destructive triumphalism over populations and over nature itself (Leonard 1979: 7). Modernity is seen as representing colonial and postcolonial domination in which the interests of Western capitalism lead to the attempted homogenization of a world of diverse cultures, beliefs and histories. Rejecting the 'master narratives' of modernity involves living with 'mininarratives' which are provisional, contingent, temporary and relative, and which provide a basis for the actions of specific groups in particular local circumstances. Rejecting totality and any claim to provide explanations for all social experience, postmodernists stress fragmentation – of language, of time, of the human subject, of society itself. In all postmodernist and poststructuralist discourses, the nature of the human subject (even sometimes its existence as a category of analysis), subjectivity and rational consciousness are put into question. This sets a serious challenge to radical welfare and educational practice which has often grounded itself in humanist accounts of human needs and human rights.

Negotiating the challenge

Is an attempt to find an accommodation between a general theory of inequality and a recognition of diversity undermined by postmodernist and poststructuralist ideas, as by, for example, Cealey Harrison and Hood-Williams (1998)? This challenge has prompted critical theorists to seek for ways in which universal values of justice and emancipation can be maintained while at the same time accepting the reality of global diversity within gender and among cultures, sexualities, abilities and ages. As Fiona Williams has argued, feminism has an important role to play in engaging this debate (Williams 1996). First, there is a tendency in poststructuralist critiques to neglect the social context and to de-emphasize economic and material relations of power. The evidence for global inequalities of gender, 'race' and class is well documented (Anthias and Yuval Davis 1992; Dalla Costa and Dalla Costa 1993; Doyal 1995; Leonard 1997; Lister 1997a; Mama 1989; Townsend 1993; UN 1991; Walby 1990, 1997). These categories are not constructed solely discursively. The evidence for the material existence of inequality is irrefutable, though it takes diverse forms and different factors may be of overriding political concern for different groups at different times and places. As Walby (1997) notes, while relations of power could potentially take an infinite number of forms, in actuality there are some widely repeated features. This insight leads Doyal (1995) to reject what she calls 'crude universalism and crude difference theories' and to posit a concept of 'common difference'. Lister (1997a) speaks of differentiated universalism, to capture the tension between the universal and the particular. Benhabib conceptualizes an 'interactive universalism' (1992: 3) to acknowledge the plurality of modes of being human. In these accounts, differences and separations do not of themselves pose a serious threat to effective political action and the possibility of theory (Sawicki 1991: 17). Feminists in particular have set about developing such theory and political action.

All the contributors to this volume share in the critique of universalizing theories which mask understanding of the impact of oppression, and all write from a recognition of the different forms oppression takes. Each contributor – including the two editors – formulates their relationship to the critique of modernity and modernist accounts differently. There are few essays here that are not influenced by the work of Foucault. Equally, there are few writers here who would reject humanist aspirations for justice, progress and emancipation and all would be concerned to have a voice in the definition of these goals.

Welfare, discipline, control and resistance

The work of Michel Foucault has made a significant contribution to an understanding and analysis of the changes which have taken place. Foucault's theory of discourse insists upon historical specificity: that is, that an analysis must look to the specific detail of the discursive field which constitutes, for example, madness, punishment or sexuality, in order to uncover the particular regimes of power and knowledge at work in a society, and their part in the overall production and maintenance of existing power relations. Discourses are ways of constituting knowledge, together with social practices, forms of subjectivity and power relations which inhere in such knowledges and the relations between them. This is always part of a wider network of power relations, often with institutional bases (Foucault 1981). Unlike the Hegelian tradition of the analysis of power, Foucault does not utilize history as a means of locating a single revolutionary subject, nor does he locate power in a single material base. His focus is on the myriad power relations that are networked throughout societies and which make centralized repressive forms of power possible. He posits a view of power as exercised rather than possessed and not primarily repressive, but productive. The analysis of discursive practices as sites of power enables an account of the way subjects are constituted by power relations.

Fraser (1989) argues that the terrain of the social is a space in which discursive and political struggles over the definition of needs occur: these include the 'expert' discourses of professionals. It is illuminating to link such a feminist analysis with analyses building on Foucauldian thinking, and on Gramscian accounts of civil society, which have become so important to much critical analysis of professional practice, and are developed by a number of contributors to this book. The concept of discursive practices which constitute power relationships and identities has drawn critical attention to particular patterns of dominance and subordination in the production of 'professional' and 'client' subject positions, and at the same time has brought recognition for subjugated voices and insurrectionary knowledges. The analysis of discourses is non-reductive; it does not seek out one underlying story, or one universal subject for the processes of human emancipation. It does, however, continually hold open the possibility of change, if not of transformation. It deflects political attention from centres of power – there is no longer one centre of power which is the focus of political activity – 'the commanding heights of the economy', 'the military', 'the broadcasting industry' – and able to be seized. Instead power is conceived of as produced in the relations of discourses: practices, networks, affiliations which are always open to reversal and contestation, always productive of challenge to their own powerful directions. The lunatics are always threatening to take over the asylum.

Not all the writers in this collection would accept the Foucauldian account of power as decentred and resistance as always localized. For some of the writers here, the state continues to be the key focus of political struggle; and it remains necessary to identify and acknowledge key global centres of economic and military power: what was once termed 'the military industrial complex' of transnational corporations and the nuclear weapons industry, whose power, while identified and resisted locally, is understood as global and will only be effectively countered globally. There are some interesting questions being developed by some writers about the connections between a Foucauldian account of power and the account of economic power, and these emphasize the role of diversification of economic power within a global market (Harvey 1989; Haraway 1991). However, for all contributors, the question of what counts as political has been transformed in our engagement with the struggles encountered in welfare practice. The political now includes debate about sexuality and family relationships, health care and schooling, therapy and psychological treatments, prisons and the criminal justice system. These are no longer conceived as apolitical matters of professional expertise, or as the outcomes of economic calculations made elsewhere. Discourses in all these areas are the sites of political contest in their own right: a contest, as Fraser (1989) puts it, of needs interpretation, and also over identities, communities and belonging.

Critical professionals

There is no such thing as a neutral professional, and never has been. Even before the New Right and New Labour notions of welfare workers as regulators of an excluded underclass, liberal education encouraged an uncritical attitude to theory. Power relations were not explicitly addressed, and the teaching of values operated in a conceptual power vacuum. As a result, 'values' has been subject to colonization in a changing political context. In social work for example, although the language of 'anti-discrimination' and 'anti-racism' has been a preoccupation of training for a number of years, from the start it was purged of its radical potential by constant redefinition and incorporation into prevailing notions of welfare practice.

If there is no such thing as a neutral professional, is professional work within state bureaucracies inevitably reactionary and supportive of the status quo? Is it possible to push our way towards 'critical intelligence' (Mayo and Thompson 1995) which will make a difference? We have coined the phrase 'critical professionals', which, though it may sound contradictory, expresses our belief that educators and practitioners can to an extent, as we have suggested above, work in the interests of their students/clients towards challenging the hegemony of the market. As Jane Thompson says, we can 'remain engaged in the process of contesting the purpose and significance of learning (and education and welfare practice), as distinct from measuring everything that moves on a five-point scale' (Thompson 1995: 4).

A key element of this is engaging with theory in a way which does not ignore the *context* within which professional practice takes place and which seeks alternatives to the technicist and instrumentalist role imposed upon professionals. Theory, seen currently as 'methods of intervention' to aid problem solving, needs to be used as a way of problematizing reality, of rendering power relations visible. The critical professional not only acknowledges subjugated knowledges but actively works to make alternative definitions of need influential in the responses to need. She also recognizes difference, not for the purpose of 'managing' diversity and deconstructing subjectivity, but as a basis for resistance against the positioning of particular identities as subordinate (Williams 1996). Crucially, she is engaged in collective action, working across differences with clients and colleagues in specific local issues towards a common goal of ending injustice. These themes are developed further in the chapter by Humphries in this volume.

At the very border created by excluding discourses and practices, new voices and reverse discourses come into being. In much welfare discourse, particularly in the discourses of professionalism, a clear-cut distinction is held to exist between the professional and the client. From one account, (Smith 1987), this can be understood as the means by which the professional class asserts its control within the system and the client/user either colludes with or resists that control. The discourses and practices of welfare are analysed as a site of struggles: a site in which the subjection of welfare dependants in a variety of forms can lead to the emergence of new voices, entering into a political dialogue about needs, rights and citizenship. Feminist analyses of the links between the personal, the social and the political have been central to the development of this understanding. The recognition that existing theorizations have effectively excluded women's perspectives from the domain of the political, subordinating them to the 'private' domain of the family, has instigated much fruitful theoretical work. Feminist analyses – among others – have opened up the possibility of dialogue between professionals and clients, in a participatory approach to the interpretation of need. While not denying the experience of class difference between professionals and users/clients, it is possible to recognize the possibility of common ground, or a shared set of non-expert knowledges, in which a critical dialogue may occur between professionals and the various user/survivor movements.

Rethinking citizenship

How do those who do not currently control the definition and interpretation of need make their presence felt in the discursive arena? In this collection of essays, we aim to develop critical thinking about the practice of welfare and to enable the development of networks and alliances between welfare professionals and clients/users which can resist the practices of welfare and education concerned merely with social reproduction and social control. We have, therefore, to turn to the question of the definition of citizenship, and the question of voice and agency.

There are clearly major limits to individualist conceptions of political authority and political agency, and yet it is from a reworking of the classical liberal accounts of the citizen and his rights that some of the most exciting work in political theory is currently occurring. Some of these reworkings take on the insights of poststructuralist theories. Human rights, for example, can be understood not as a possession of citizens, but as dialectical and relational in opening up debates about how to alter relationships of oppression positively. Human rights are seen as dialogical rights, 'predicated fundamentally on the right to give voice and be listened to in the process of decision making' (Yeatman 1994: 90).

Citizenship matters because it can act as a powerful exclusionary device – no citizenship, no entitlement – and conversely, in liberal democracies, it provides the grounds of entry on to the terrain of the political. There are two strong and distinct accounts of citizenship available within conventional political theory: the liberal tradition which associates citizenship with status and the possession of rights, and the civic republican tradition which associates citizenship with a much more active participation in the pursuit of the good for a particular community. Feminist debate is currently transforming both these definitions of citizenship, and Ruth Lister has recently argued that in this transformation it is the concept of human agency which is central (Lister 1997a). In defining citizenship we are seeking the conditions which will enable participation in the political sphere and therefore enable us to act as subjects and agents in our own lives, and not as passive objects of the charity of others.

Lister argues that, although formed in different conceptual frameworks, the liberal and republican traditions are not incompatible, but that both need to be transformed by the insights of those excluded from the forum.

> Citizenship as participation represents an expression of human agency in the political arena, broadly defined; citizenship as rights enables people to act as agents. Moreover, citizenship rights are not fixed. They remain the object of political struggles to define, reinterpret and extend them.
>
> (Lister 1997b: 35)

In other words, the redefinition of citizenship and rights and the redefinition of the content of political debate go hand in hand. The entry of women's voices into political debate has begun to extend concepts of human rights into discussion of reproductive rights and of freedom from violence in intimate relationships, for example. It also challenges the exclusion of unpaid labour from citizenship entitlement, and looks for compatibility between paid work and caring, and structures that will help people to share unpaid work. What else would become central to political debate if the voices of prisoners, asylum seekers, lone parents, lesbian mothers, children excluded from school, were able to be present in political debate on their own behalf?

Welfare, voice and agency

Much theoretical work in this area has developed a positive account of the possibility of 'reverse discourses' and the voicing of subjugated and insurrectionary knowledges. But at the same time, in the critique of the human subject as the source of authority, authorship and power, and in the understanding of that subject as an effect of discursive practices, there has been a deathly evacuation of a sense of political agency. For both professionals and clients in search of resources of hope which can undermine the oppressive practices, an account of potential sources of change is vital.

If, as some postmodernist and poststructuralist accounts suggest, the liberal individual as the source of political action has died and if there are no consistently identifiable sources of collective power from which to challenge hegemonic discursive practices, then the prospects for excluded groups seem bleak, unless occasional raiding and sabotaging can effect a more consistent reversal. It is for this reason that concepts of voice, dialogue and agency have become so central to our thinking as the work for this book has developed. We want to continue to work in that tradition, articulated in its masculinist form by Marx: 'Men [and women] make their own history, but they do not make it just as they please; they do not make it under circumstances chosen by themselves, but under circumstances directly encountered, given and transmitted from the past' (Marx 1968: 97).

The concept of 'voice' and 'agency' involves far more than is usually considered in relation to welfare as 'good practice' in promoting participation and user involvement in the management of services. It is important for welfare professionals to consider how best to engage with powerful perspectives emerging in organized form from groups who have not so far defined the nature of 'good practice'. Power has been exercised in welfare practice by claims to knowledge which are abstract, generalizable, universal. Many of these scientific claims to knowledge have been incorporated – via medicine and psychology in particular – into welfare discourse. In this context, the claim to knowledge about others is a claim to power in relation to them, for good or ill. The power lies in part in the capacity to define, analyse and name – even bring into being – human populations, and to establish, through these claims to knowledge, systems of control of those populations.

Within any discursive practice, however, there have been ways of knowing that are subjugated. In producing new subjects and new possibilities of social relationship, discursive practices also produce new possibilities of knowledge. If criminology produces an account of the pathologically violent criminal, it also produces the possibility of that same criminal authorizing his own account of violence. When educational psychology produces evidence of the behaviours on account of which a pupil should be excluded from school, it produces the possibility of that pupil voicing her/his own account. Sexology produces the subject position of the 'homosexual', and lesbians talk back, problematizing the same discourses which render lesbian existence problematic. This 'talking back' occurs in cultural work and in the communications industry as well as in academe and in new and emerging welfare organizations. It is to these voices with power behind them that, we are arguing, critical welfare professionals need to be attentive.

The importance of testimony – of speaking individually and/or within a community – on our own behalf, has been central to a number of the new social and political movements. It has been particularly important in those communities where the experience of discrimination and exclusion has been linked to subjectification and the assignation of identity. Humanist perspectives which authorize the individual and the speaking subject remain very important here, and the critique of humanism associated with Althusser and Foucault has failed to grapple thoroughly with the question of the sources of authority and power available to oppressed and marginalized peoples. The idea of agency is more than individual. Humans are social from the start. Social relations are essential to individual development, and we characteristically engage in common activities, oriented to common and not merely individual ends. Political agency means finding ways of making common cause out of those shared ends, entering into dialogue about shared and different interests and needs The negotiation of the groups with whom common cause is made is not a natural process, but a discursive cultural process and a profoundly political one. In Nira Yuval Davis' (1994) theorizations, these processes, for citizens challenging current hegemonic discourses, involve the formation of 'transversal alliances', dialogic networks embodying practices of 'rooting' and 'shifting'. In such alliances, participants remain rooted in their own identities and values but are willing to shift their views in dialogue with others. We hope that the chapters in this book will contribute to the formation of such 'transversal alliances' between critical professionals and clients/users, which will challenge the monological practice of juridical, technical and administrative discourses which dominate welfare practice currently.

The themes we have explored in this chapter are emphasized in a variety of ways in the chapters which follow. Early chapters are particularly concerned with the role of welfare in the process of exclusion, in defining 'them' and 'us', citizens and non-citizens, and with the pivotal role of legacies of nineteenth-century internal control of the poor and the impact of the 'return effect' of empire. Tom Cockburn demonstrates how the treatment of children and their exclusion from citizenship formed the ground of contemporary patterns of welfare in which professional power to control and protect is so pronounced. Daryl Crosskill analyses contemporary colonial patterns in Sir Roy Griffiths' formation of policy on 'community care'. 'The poor' have replaced 'the native' as the objects of colonial disciplinary strategies, with professionals, as 'care managers', positioned as the petty-officers of that power, in contrast with the care workers – often YTS trainees or other low-paid workers – who are 'the people who are in direct contact with the users of services and in some sense share their status'. The place of policy in enabling such exclusions and in shaping a politics of needs interpretation is made clear.

Debra Hayes also highlights the centrality of the legacies of imperialist nationalism and racism in welfare, showing how discourses of 'scarce resources' and 'the health of the nation' are critical in the separation of the deserving and the undeserving, and particularly in the harsh treatment offered to asylum seekers and refugees. Again, the potential solidarity between some of the lowest paid workers in health and welfare and those on the receiving end of racist and exclusionary practices is highlighted.

The question of potential solidarities between those located as 'professionals' and their 'clients' – and of whether the concept of 'critical professionals' which we have debated in this chapter has any purchase in practice – is highlighted in a variety of ways in the next chapters. Gill Aitken introduces the debate among white professionals about the impact of racism in psychological services, and how those services have been shaped by racialized assumptions to which they have remained blind in the name of science and professional person-centred approaches. Mary Issitt investigates what has happened to feminist politics in welfare, as a result of the impact of the marketization of services and the development of a 'competence culture' in training. Vic Tuck highlights the ways in which pathologizing of 'cycles of deprivation' and of family violence can disguise the impact of poverty, depoliticizing family social work and leading to a reluctance on the part of social workers to join in anti-poverty movements. In a similar way, Carol Packham highlights the contradictory nature of current education policies, which create the problem of exclusion they then set out to solve. She shows how the exclusion of the young black male has become a focus of political attention, distracting from wider debates about the purpose of education, the informal exclusion of other, perhaps more 'docile' populations, and the question of what an inclusive education system would offer. Beth Humphries sees potential in international alliances among welfare workers to offer resources of hope, as well as in an emphasis on a wider basis of knowledge and understanding than that offered by technicist and competence-based models of education.

In the last three chapters, the question of enabling the voice and agency of those who are excluded from dominant 'expert' knowledges is addressed. The challenge (and the potential limitations) of user movements in relation to self-harm are explored by Helen Spandler and Janet Batsleer, in a chapter which also acknowledges the importance of popular cultural forms – in this case music – in any discussion of voice and agency.

The potential of autobiography as a form to challenge dominant constructions of criminality and masculinity, including black masculinity, is explored by Steve Morgan, in his discussion of three prisoners' stories. And Helen Williamson uses research interviews as a method of giving voice to and rendering visible the diversity of lesbian experiences of 'coming out', and of lesbian agency in the assessment of risk from the dominant heterosexual culture.

It is clear that the chapters which follow cannot be read as pursuing a single line of argument. However, the connections between them are evident. We are seeking to rekindle a sense of political analysis and of political agency among welfare professionals, which might be stronger than the vacuous talk about 'values' and 'identities' which we have lived with for too long. We hope to facilitate dialogue which will restore a sense of political agency among those who have most at stake in challenging current oppressive relationships and practices, and thus not just to theorize difference but to contribute to the mediation of those differences in shaping the direction of social policy and welfare practice for the future.

References

Alexander, D. and Martin, I. (1995) 'Competence, curriculum and democracy', in M. Mayo and J. Thompson (eds), *Adult Learning, Critical Intelligence and Social Change*, Leicester: National Institute of Adult Continuing Education, 69–96.

Amos, V. and Parmar, P. (1984) 'Challenging imperialist feminism', *Feminist Review*, 17, 3–19.

Anthias, F. and Yuval Davis, N. (1992) *Racialized Boundaries*, London and New York: Routledge.

Benhabib, S. (1992) *Situating the Self*, Cambridge: Polity Press.

Bowlby, J. (1953) *Childcare and the Growth of Love*, Harmondsworth: Penguin.

Carabine, J. (1996) 'Heterosexuality and social policy', in D. Richardson (ed.), *Theorising Heterosexuality*, Buckingham: Open University Press, 55–74.

Carby, H.V. (1982) 'White woman listen! Black feminism and the boundaries of sisterhood', in Centre for Contemporary Cultural Studies, *The Empire Strikes Back*, London: Hutchinson, 212–35.

Cealey Harrison, W. and Hood-Williams, J. (1998) 'More varieties than Heinz: social categories and sociality in Humphries, Hammersley and beyond', *Sociological Research Online*, 3 (1), http://www.socresonline.org.uk/socresonline/3/1/8.html

Clarke, J. (1996) 'After social work?' in N. Parton (ed.), *Social Theory, Social Change and Social Work*, London: Routledge.

Dalla Costa, M. and Dalla Costa, G. (eds), (1993) *Paying the Price*, London and New Jersey: Zed Books.

Dominelli, L. (1991) *Women Across Continents*, Hemel Hempstead: Harvester Wheatsheaf.

Doyal, L. (1995)*What Makes Women Sick: Gender and the Political Economy of Health*, London: Macmillan.

Edwards, R. and Usher, R. (1994) 'Disciplining the subject: the power of competence', *Studies in the Education of Adults*, 26 (1), 1–14.

Esping-Andersen, G. (ed.) (1996) *Welfare States in Transition*, London: Sage.

Foucault, M. (1981) *The History of Sexuality, Vol. 1: An Introduction*, Harmondsworth: Pelican.

Fraser, N. (1989) 'Women, welfare and the politics of needs interpretation' in P. Lassman (ed.), *Politics and Social Theory*, London: Routledge.

Graham, H. (1993) *Hardship and Health in Women's Lives*, New York, London: Harvester Wheatsheaf.

Hammar, T. (1990) *Democracy and the Nation State*, Aldershot: Avebury.

Haraway, D. (1991) *Simians, Cyborgs and Women: The Reinvention of Science*, New York: Routledge.

Harding, S. (1991) *Whose Science? Whose Knowledge? Thinking from Women's Lives*, Milton Keynes: Open University Press.

Harvey, D. (1989) *The Condition of Postmodernity*, Oxford: Blackwell.

hooks, b. (1982) *Ain't I a Woman? Black Women and Feminism*, London: Pluto Press.

Humphries, B. (1997) 'Reading social work: competing discourses in the Rules and Requirements for the Diploma in Social Work', *British Journal of Social Work* 27 (5), 641–58.

Jones, C. (1996) 'Anti-intellectualism and social work education', in N. Parton (ed.), *Social Theory, Social Change and Social Work*, London, New York: Routledge, 190–210.

Jones, C. and Novak, T. (1993) 'Social Work Today', *British Journal of Social Work*, 23 (2): 195–212.

Leonard, P. (1979) *Postmodern Welfare,* London: Sage.

Levitas, R. (1996) 'The concept of social exclusion and the new Durkheimian hegemony', *Critical Social Policy*, 46, 16, 5–20.

Lewis, G. (1996) 'Situated voices: black women's experience and social work', *Feminist Review*, 53, 24–56.

Lister, R. (1997a) *Citizenship: feminist perspectives*, London: Macmillan.

——(1997b) 'Citizenship: towards a feminist synthesis', in *Feminist Review* 57, 28–48.

Lorde, A. (1984) *Sister Outsider*, New York: The Crossing Press.

Lyotard, J.F. (1979) *The Postmodern Condition: A Report on Knowledge*, Manchester: Manchester University Press.

Mama, A. (1989) *The Hidden Struggle*, London: Race and Housing Research Unit and Runnymede Trust.

Marshall, T.H. (1950) *Citizenship and Social Class and Other Essays*, Cambridge: Cambridge University Press.

Marx, K. (1968) [1852] 'The Eighteenth Brumaire of Louis Bonaparte', in K. Marx and F. Engels, *Selected Works*, London: Lawrence and Wishart.

Mayo, M. and Thompson, J. (eds) (1995) *Adult Learning, Critical Intelligence and Social Change*, Leicester: National Association of Adult Continuing Education.

Mead, L. (1986) *Beyond Entitlement: The Social Obligations of Citizenship*, New York: The Free Press.

Mohanty, C. T. (1991) 'Under western eyes: feminist scholarship and colonial discourses', in C.T. Mohanty, A. Russo and L. Torres (eds), *Third World Women and the Politics of Feminism*, Indianapolis: Indiana University Press, 51–80.

Muncie, J. and Sparks, R. (eds) (1991) *Imprisonment, European Perspectives*, New York, London: Harvester Wheatsheaf.

Novak, M. (1987) *A Community of Self-Reliance: The New Consensus on Family and Welfare*, Milwaukee: American Enterprise Institute for Public Policy Research.

Oppenheim, C. and Harper, L. (1996) *Poverty: The Facts*, London: Child Poverty Action Group.

Pascall, G. (1997) *Social Policy: A New Feminist Analysis*, London: Routledge.
Price, J. (1996) 'The marginal politics of our bodies? Women's health, the disability movement, and power', in B. Humphries (ed.), *Critical Perspectives on Empowerment*, Birmingham: Venture Press, 35–52.
Sawicki, J. (1991) *Disciplining Foucault: Feminism, Power and the Body*, New York, London: Routledge.
Sibley, D. (1995) *Geographies of Exclusion: Society and Difference in the West*, London: Routledge.
Smith, D. (1987) *Social Work and the Sociology of Organisations*, London: Routledge.
Thompson, J. (1995) 'Preface', in M. Mayo and J. Thompson (eds), *Adult Learning, Critical Intelligence and Social Change*, Leicester: National Association of Adult Continuing Education, 1–4.
Townsend, P. (1993) *The International Analysis of Poverty*, New York, London: Harvester Wheatsheaf.
United Nations (1991) 'The World's Women 1970–1990: Trends and Statistics', *Social Statistics and Indicators, Series K, No. 8*, New York: UN.
Walby, S. (1990) *Theorizing Patriarchy*, Oxford: Blackwell.
——(1997) *Gender*, London, New York: Routledge.
Williams, F. (1989) *Social Policy: A Critical Introduction*, Cambridge: Polity Press.
——(1996) 'Postmodernism, feminism and the question of difference', in N. Parton (ed.), *Social Theory, Social Change and Social Work*, London: Routledge.
Yeatman, A. (1994) *Postmodern Revisionings of the Political*, London: Routledge.
Yuval Davis, N. (1994) 'Women, ethnicity and empowerment', *Feminism and Psychology*, 4 (1), 179–97.

2 From 'street arabs' to 'angels': working-class children, competence and citizenship, 1850–1914

Tom Cockburn

Introduction

Today children are in an almost unequivocal position of dependence in British society. There is a rigid formal age–class hierarchy that permeates the whole of society and creates a distance between adults and children. Special forms of dress, games, languages and attitudes sustain the status, which distances childhood from adult society. They are the subjects of an enormous weight of surveillance, monitoring, supervision, control and exclusion from adult society. They are also alleged not to be rational or capable of making reasonable decisions, lack wisdom of experience and are prone to mistakes or danger.

This view contrasts with earlier historical representations of children who were represented as 'little adults', with no singularly defining features. Debates around childhood have been deeply influenced by the work of Philippe Aries (1960) who argued that there was no concept of childhood in medieval society. Throughout the seventeenth century people began treating their children differently. Adults began treating children as playthings, seeing them as both innocent and weak, and in need of specific training and treatment different to those of adults. While the boldness of Aries' arguments about the 'discovery' of childhood has been tempered by Pollock (1983), among others (such as Wilson 1980; Jordanova 1989), who emphasizes the complexity of definitions and constructions of childhood through time and across social classes. There is a broad sense of agreement that parenthood, childhood and childcare are socially constructed in different and diverse ways throughout history (Anderson 1980). This is not to deny the effects of physical being or the importance of the biological dimension of children in their lives. Instead, the historicity of our categories should be recognized and the 'relationship between conceptual thought, social action and the process of category construction and, therefore, definitions of childhood must to some extent be dependent upon the society from which they emerge' (Hendrick 1990: 36). For instance, through recollections of working-class people themselves, we know that many children made significant financial contributions to the domestic economy through work (T. Thompson 1981; Jamieson 1986; P. Thompson 1975; F. Thompson 1945). It was also widely culturally accepted in the working-class textile districts of Lancashire and Yorkshire that children would make substantial contributions to the family's income (Steedman 1992). Many migrants to Britain in the nineteenth century expected their children to contribute to the household economy. For example, Behlmer (1982) discusses the *padrone* system, common in Italian families, and the conflicts this brought with the middle-class child protectors. While acknowledging the complexity and local variability of categories and constructions there can, nevertheless, be distinct shifts of emphases noticed in textual representations. Furthermore, these representations were real in that they impinged upon, and deeply affected, the day-to-day activities of child welfare workers.

In this chapter I illustrate shifts in categorical meanings of children, beginning with a construction of what Hendrick (1990) calls 'street children', literally children living on the streets, suffering from cold, hunger, starvation and mistreatment. The response to this newly perceived social problem was largely in terms of religious rhetoric and ideology. Action took the form of establishing missions, soup kitchens, relief projects, rescue sorties and the establishment of refuges.

The second half of this chapter discusses the effects of these discourses on children through an examination of children's position relating to citizenship. I argue that in the nineteenth century, children were gradually excluded from all realms of public life and located within clearly defined and closely controlled private spaces of the home and school. Their exclusion from citizenship was premised upon piecemeal erosion of children's competence in public life. The activities of the state over the period considered here, while enabling children to gain some autonomy over their parents, only reconstituted the image of childhood as a time of dependence, irresponsibility and, at best, 'citizens in the making'. The very justifications of acting on behalf of children as innocent objects in dire need of protection, while protecting children from abuse, further eroded their ability to take control of their own lives.

The discovery of the 'street child'

Carolyn Steedman's (1992) review of Margaret McMillan's work at the turn of the century and John Ruskin's *Fairyland,* published in 1884, emphasized the environmental location of children as a cause for concern. Ruskin and McMillan depicted working-class childhood as a symbol of beauty within the ugly, corrupting and decaying city land-scapes. The picture of what Peter Coveney (1968) describes as the romantic, post-Wordsworthian child as the embodiment of beauty and innocence, being an 'already-thwarted possibility' (Steedman 1992: 34) was a powerful image that pervaded much of the contemporary commentary on childhood. These depictions of children in hostile and corrupting conditions were in the context of wider concerns about the effects of the physical environment of the city on the urban poor.

Reformers were concerned about the environment in which children lived and worked – from at least the debates around Poor Law reform and early campaigns of factory reform in the early nineteenth century (Hopkins 1994) and medical concerns, such as James Kay's in Manchester, over the conditions of children living in slum conditions (Mort 1987). Concerns of the 'exposure' of working-class children to the corruption of the city were a continuing theme throughout the century. In the 1840s Henry Mayhew's articles for the *Morning Chronicle* (reprinted 1985) paid attention to the effects of the environ-ment on working-class children: 'Every Londoner must have seen numbers of ragged, sickly, and ill-fed children, squatting at the entrance of miserable courts, streets and alleys, engaged in no occupa-tion that is either creditable to themselves or useful to the community' (Mayhew 1985: 19).

The corruption of the urban streets, the threat of contagion from criminals, the analogies of working-class 'tribes' and 'savages', rever-berate through the pages of Mayhew's text. In 1848 Lord Ashley, veteran campaigner for factory reform, referred to more than 30,000 'naked, filthy, roaming, lawless, and deserted children, in and about the metropolis'; Edwin Chadwick warned of such children's 'perpetual tendency to moral as well as physical deterioration' (Floud and Wachter 1982). In 1840 police in Manchester reported that 3,650 chil-dren were sleeping rough in the city (Hewitt 1979: 64). In the 1850s, in poor districts in English cities (such as the Deansgate district of Manchester), the streets were perceived to be disproportionately full of starving, unhealthy and unruly children beyond middle-class reforming influences.

The large number of children wandering the streets inspired a great deal of literature about the plight of children in English cities. For instance, Elizabeth Barrett Browning's *The Cry of the Children* portrayed a grinding picture of children's lives, as did Charles Dickens' *Oliver Twist* and James Greenwood's *The Little Raggamuffins*, to name a few.

Crucially, the children were portrayed as being 'incompetent' to deal with such surroundings. Thus reformers increasingly identified children's exposure to the city streets as an object of concern needing attention. So worried were campaigners for 'street children' that many began programmes seeking to remove children from city streets, often permanently.

Margaret May (1973) has shown how concern with street children arose not entirely out of humane benevolence: there were also fears about the protection of private property. Middle-class reformers feared that children, deprived of proper moral instruction, would become trained as criminals, drunks and debauchers. The perceived increase in crime, as well as the expressed indifference towards religion and morality, motivated the establishment of Ragged School Unions in 1844 under the presidency of Lord Ashley.[1] These schools catered for the poorest sections of the population where no other provision of education existed. It also is perhaps no accident that the establishment of Ragged Schools coincided with the political agitation associated with Chartism. Elaine Hadley (1990) notes that the use of such language as 'savages', 'guttersnipes' or 'street arabs' expressed the anxieties that these children offered to an orderly society. Such language was in stark contrast to the 'innocent,' 'obedient' and 'silent' representations of children in middle-class households.

Fears over children's perceived vulnerability on the street provided the impetus for the formation of a large number of organizations 'rescuing' children from the streets. Such organizations included Barnardos, the Waifs and Strays Society, the Catholic and Jewish Rescue Societies, the Manchester and Salford Boys' and Girls' Welfare Society (known locally as the 'Manchester Refuges'),[2] numerous Methodist street-children's missions and the NSPCC, among others. Most of these organizations' primary aim was to rescue children from the 'dark dangers' that the city streets posed and to restore the young's 'natural' innocent sensibilities.

The corrupting influences of the urban environment were dealt with at the most extreme through the encouragement of emigration. Emigration appealed to many, such as the Manchester Refuges and the Catholic and Methodist Rescue Societies, as it offered prospects of employment in a healthy environment, where there was a demand for labour in a rural life far from the malignant conditions of English cities. There was no legal way institutions could force parents or guardians to allow their children to emigrate, although persuasion and encouragement of emigration were successfully used by most child welfare organizations from the middle of the nineteenth century. Other charitable organizations used emigration schemes, such as those of the Salvation Army and the Jewish Board of Guardians in Manchester. The policy of emigration for institutionalized children continued up to 1967 (Bean and Melville 1989: 28). Between 1860 and 1920, 90,000 children were exported from Britain to Canada alone (Bean and Melville 1989: 20).

Mary Carpenter, in her tireless campaigns for a more generous understanding of offending children, argued for a new approach to dealing with children. In her numerous writings she argued that only with love, compassion, understanding and care can children be truly reformed. In the 1880s there was a consciously religious-inspired depiction of street children being 'rescued' from the corrupting environment of the city slum (Cunningham 1991). Indicating the potential within the individual for redemption, the Religious Tract Society published Hesba Stretton's *Jessica's First Prayer*, *Pilgrim Street* and *A Tale of Manchester Life*. Alfred Alsop, the superintendent of the Wood Street Mission[3] in Manchester, produced a number of popular tracts under the name of A. Delver. The stories were popular enough that the publishers claimed that each volume sold about 30,000 copies (Thomas 1985: 207).[4] The stories were produced both to raise funds for the Wood Street Mission and to develop middle-class consciousness about the plight of street children.[5] In one of the stories, called 'Little Boz', the boy character came from a home where he was beaten by a drunken mother. The boy, found by one of the mission workers cold and hungry and selling newspapers, was admitted to the shelter and placed in an Industrial School and sailed happily to Canada. The narratives consisted of themes of a childhood lost and a childhood redeemed. The stories, it was hoped, would convince the reader that street children were redeemable and that the institutions could utilize their knowledge and skills to reform their characters.

From the mid-nineteenth century the state became increasingly involved in various aspects of children's lives, replacing a number of welfare, educational and social functions previously provided by voluntary bodies. The state also began to intervene in what had previously been believed to be the 'private' world of the family. The state, as in earlier legislation to curtail children's employment in factories (Cunningham 1987), intervened to act *in loco parentis* where parents

were failing to provide for the physical, mental and moral welfare of
their offspring. The major 'failure' of parents was to allow their children to wander the streets. The 1868 Industrial Schools Act permitted
that

> any person may bring before two justices or a magistrate any child
> apparently under the age of fourteen years that comes within any
> of the following descriptions, namely: That is found begging or
> receiving alms ... that is found wandering ... that is, found desti-
> tute ... that frequents the company of reputed thieves.
>
> (quoted in Pugh 1980: 8)

The passing of the 1868 Industrial Schools Act resulted in the
provision of a number of Industrial Schools, such as the well-reputed
Manchester schools in Ardwick and Monsall and the already existing
Swinton School. In 1877 the Manchester School Board appointed four
officers to report on the progress of children leaving the schools. They
also found homeless children positions as apprentices to become
colliers or farmers or, in the case of girls, found positions for them in
domestic service (6th Annual Report of the Manchester Local
Government Board, 1877). The justification for the existence of
Industrial Schools was based on the idea that children be 'completely
severed from associates and localities of a degrading and demoralising
character' (National Association for the Promotion of Social Science
(NAPSS) 1884: 224).[6] Captain J. Rowland Brookes, Superintendent of
the Middlesex Industrial School, argued that when children were

> removed from all previous surroundings, and too often from the
> bad example of pernicious parents, an opportunity is afforded
> them of acquiring habits of honesty and industry, which, being
> supplemented by religious teaching, gradually enables the children
> to form correct ideas of moral rectitude and of their duty to God
> and their neighbour.
>
> (NAPSS 1884: 225)

By the First World War the number of children roaming the streets
had fallen dramatically and the 'street child' was no longer a powerful
symbolic image. Thomas Ackroyd of the Manchester Refuges boasted
in 1914,

> I may say that I could not now take you to a single place in
> Manchester and Salford where a child can be found sleeping out

and, speaking with a very wide experience of other centres, I can say emphatically that in no city approaching the size of Manchester are there fewer ragged and destitute children. It is now a rare sight to discover anything approaching the old type of street Arab. This I attribute very largely to the splendid philanthropic agencies which have been at work in our midst for many years.

(*Manchester Evening Chronicle*, 16 February 1914)

It seems, however, that this was due perhaps less to philanthropic endeavour than to a combination of developments in educational and welfare services discussed below, the falling birth and infant mortality rates,[7] and the determined efforts of the Manchester Corporation and the Manchester police to prohibit all street trading by children without a licence.[8] No licence was granted to any child under 12 years old, nor any girl under 14, and all street trading by children was prohibited after nine o'clock. Manchester Corporation's policy of controlling child street trading is fully discussed in Cockburn (1992).

The erosion of children's competence and citizenship

Given that children today have little or no independent civil, political and social rights, and yet it is as children that people are defined, trained, prepared, protected and categorized for their future roles as citizens, it is necessary to investigate the relationship between children and citizenship. For this it is more appropriate to look at that period of time when citizenship was extended and defined in England, in the nineteenth and early twentieth centuries.

Middle-class ideals of femininity in the nineteenth century have been associated by Davidoff and Hall (1988) with a 'childlike' vulnerability, an incomplete and under-developed nature which was hence socially dependent and in need of protection. The feminist critique of this ideology argues that such qualities are not specific 'natures' but a socially constructed ideology that served to maintain the patriarchal domination of women by men (e.g. Gorham 1982). While women and children were linked in their social dependency, women came to be characterized as inferior as a result of their sexual biology, while Viviana Zelizer (1985) notes that children were de-sexed into a gender-free zone of innocence, or 'sacralized'.

This sacralization was an ongoing process through the nineteenth century and applied to working-class children through definitions in Royal Commissions, social commentary and the 'revelations' by Stead that prompted a purity campaign to raise the age of consent for girls from 13 to 16. The revelations composed the exposure of child prostitution, white slavery, kidnapping, the buying and selling of children and sexual exploitation of young children by a dissolute aristocracy (Gorham 1982; Cockburn 1992). Children's 'innocence' was perceived to be in need of protection and children became subjects for a host of discourses and organizations acting 'on behalf of children' or 'in their best interests'. In a similar way that women in the early part of the nineteenth century were denied the basic rights of citizenship, such as the ownership of property and the vote, children were stripped of the means to act on their own behalf and to control the circumstances in which they found themselves. It must not be forgotten that these changes occurred in the historical context of a feminist movement challenging previous relations between both men and women and adults and children.

In the course of the passing of the Criminal Law Amendment Act of 1885, children's 'sacrilization' was officially defined and a minimum age of consent pronounced. The basic provision of the bill was the raising of the age of consent for a girl to 16; also, brothels could be searched on the basis of a sworn statement by any parent, guardian or someone acting in the *bona fide* interests of a missing girl in front of a magistrate; young girls could be removed from immoral parents; action could be taken against anybody procuring a girl under 16 or any woman by force; all 'idiot' and 'imbecile' females were singled out for protection (*Hansard*, August 1885: 1553). Parliament also passed an amendment by the Radical MP Henry Labouchere, making illegal all procurements or attempts at procurement of males for public or private indecency. The Labouchere amendment was added almost without a murmur of dissent, being passed late at night with little publicity or lobbying. Jeffrey Weeks (1977) situates this amendment in the light of a sharpening definition and hostility towards homosexuality both in Britain and abroad (Weeks 1977: 15). It was situated in a crop of sexual scandals in boys' public schools in the 1880s and the perception that homosexuality, if unchecked would 'corrupt' the nation's youth. These again resurfaced in the Cleveland Street scandal of 1889–90, involving prominent aristocrats, telegraph boys, a homosexual brothel and a son of the Prince of Wales (Weeks 1977: 19) and in 1895 with the trial of Oscar Wilde.

Purity campaigns for more stringent legislation over public displays of sexuality coincided with alarm in middle-class circles about the immorality of the unrespectable poor, or the 'residuum' (Stedman Jones 1984, chapters 9–13). In 1883 Andrew Mearns, a London Congregationalist minister, wrote the pamphlet *The Bitter Cry of*

Outcast London, exposing moral corruption and absolute godlessness in the centre of London. Mearns argued, to a receptive middle-class audience, that overcrowding in poor districts spread the infection of immorality from the dissolute to honest and upright working-class families. The next year an extensive survey, the *Report of the Royal Commission on the Housing of the Working Classes, 1884*, investigated the appalling overcrowding of working-class housing which, according to some of the investigators including Mearns, resulted in incest. The crowded bedrooms encouraged children to be sexually aware of physical matters from an early age, and it was feared that this 'corruption' of children would be detrimental to the long-term morality of the nation.

The contradictions in the need to protect and control children can be seen in the two prevailing and almost totally opposite images of children in the late nineteenth century. The first is what Peter Coveney (1968) calls the 'post-Wordsworthian child' in literature from the 1830s onwards, where the child is endowed with romantic, pristine and angelic qualities. The other is the 'non-child' of the East End gutters, the northern mills, and the child worker, conflicting with the bourgeois ideal of childhood as a separate and delicate stage in a person's life (Cunningham 1987). The campaigns around child protection can be seen as the appropriation of working-class children to conformity to middle-class ideals. With regard to the 'Maiden Tribute' revelations, the construction of the 'innocent' working-class child occurred in relation to the 'corrupted' white slave. Stead and his allies perceived danger to sexually innocent children and campaigned for the state to intervene in a more vigorous way to protect working-class minors. They also sought to extend the official and legal category of sexual innocence, especially for girls, from the age of 13 to 16. The work of 'professionalizing' agencies such as the NSPCC, Barnardos and provincial child protection agencies, occurred in the background of the campaign. These organizations from the 1880s became increasingly involved in policies in relation to children, as a separate social and legal category, in terms of their 'expertise' regarding (in)appropriate childish behaviour and behaviour towards children.

Children were also starting to be considered as 'in need of' education. In similar ways working-class people were beginning to be seen by the middle classes as unable to act responsibly unless they were taught to be so, and it was perceived that if working people were to be given rights to citizenship then a system of education was necessary to 'instruct' them on how to best use this citizenship. Compulsory mass education was enforced in the period after the 1870 Education Act.

The 1880 Mundella Act introduced compulsory school attendance between the ages of 5 and 10, with parents being responsible for sending their children to school. The 1880 Act also established School Attendance Committees to formulate and enforce bylaws. The numbers of children on the registers of inspected schools rose from 1 million in 1870 to 6 million in 1900. According to the 1851 census, only 54 per cent of 5 to 15 year olds attended school; by 1901 it was reported that 91.5 per cent attended schools regularly.

Education systems do not grow up by mere chance; they reflect contemporary ideas about social organization, the nature of knowledge, and the possibility of human improvement and notions of citizenship. Nineteenth century England saw the development of a 'universalized' structure of education for every child: every child, by the end of the century, was legally obliged to attend some formal schooling. The exact nature of this formal education was conditioned by a wide range of social factors including age, class, gender, religion, ethnicity or locality; and each of these was in the process of changing, given the large shift in social understandings of and attitudes towards them over the course of the century, and the complex interrelationship between them. Such shifting complexities affected conceptions of childhood and children, and attitudes and beliefs about the natures of children and childhood affected the types of education available within a society at any one time.

Throughout the nineteenth century, attitudes to knowledge were changing; traditionally, knowledge, especially for working-class people, was transmitted through practice and experience, often from father to son and mother to daughter in face-to-face interaction. However, the new view that knowledge could be transmitted secondarily through books and teaching and was distinct from experience was gradually being accepted (Musgrave 1968: 58). There was also a belief, increasingly taken up by industrialists, that scientific and technical education was crucial if Britain was to retain her competitiveness in the world market, in particular noticing the educational reforms in the USA and Germany (Taunton Commission 1864–8). Since the English industrial revolution, the system of long apprenticeships into trades was declining, and schooling was seen as a necessary substitute. Employers hoped that the people would be schooled into a sober and industrious workforce. This was reflected in the clutch of Committees and Commissions set up by the government; these included the Samuelson Select Committee on Scientific Instruction of 1867–8, and the Royal Commissions on Technical Instruction of 1870–5 and 1881–4.

Notions of 'reason' and 'science' were not replacing religious values;

rather religion was itself changing and becoming more complex. Since the foundation of the Society for Promoting Christian Knowledge in the eighteenth century, evangelical religion played an important role in attempting to provide some schooling for every child in the country. It was felt by a large number of evangelists that education could be used in a rehabilitative way by 'reclaiming' working-class children, and Ragged Schools were established in most towns in England. In the early nineteenth century a clutch of nonconformist schools opened for fee-paying middle-class children, such as the Congregationalist School in Mill Hill, London, in 1907 and the Society of Friends School in York in 1813.

Another change in the nineteenth century was the shifting notion and composition of 'citizenship'. The feminist movement, from Mary Wollstonecraft in the eighteenth century on, argued for a change in the relationship between men and women, the means for economic independence for women, and an improved educational provision for women and girls – if not on equal terms with boys and men then superior to it (Spender 1987: 6). Educational equality was seen by middle-class feminists to be a first step or a key to other freedoms such as access to employment opportunities, the relief of boredom and an increased ability to fight for other freedoms, and an equivalent right to citizenship with men. Second, some working-class leaders felt that education was a beneficial provision, both as a necessity in itself and as a means to social mobility (Hurt 1979). Such 'moral force' socialists, such as the Chartist William Lovett, founded adult schools, debating clubs and libraries. This commitment to a policy of educational importance was retained through the Fabian era and the post World War I Labour Party.

The upper and working classes gradually warmed to the idea of educational expansion as a means to ensure social discipline. With the urbanization of cities and the perceived threat of possible unrest, education, it was hoped, could be aimed at the children of the poor who could be provided with instruction into knowing one's place in the social hierarchy. Against the social contagion of subversive doctrines such as radicalism and anarchism, children would be made into pillars of the establishment. Through the nineteenth century the idea of 'liberalism' was changing from Whiggish laissez-faire arguments to the idealist philosophy associated with T.H. Green. Green developed a notion of citizenship based on justice, equality, middle-class values and a quest for self-help and moral improvement, and conceived of education as the great social harmonizer and equalizer of both men and women, rich and poor.

The 1888 Royal Commission on Elementary Education occurred in the historical context of the changing meanings attached to education, where the processes of vocational education and instruction to citizenship were as important as 'liberal' notions of education being beneficial in itself. Discussions surrounding the Royal Commission included the denominational disputes about the distribution of souls and over the religious instruction of children, and this illustrates the powerful beliefs those religious leaders held concerning the power and importance of education. Similarly, socialists and feminists perceived education as important to the development of liberated, responsible and independent men and women. Christian Socialists such as F.D. Maurice understood that campaigns for educational provision could not be separated from other campaigns such as co-operative production.

At the beginning of the nineteenth century, formal educational provision was very limited for working-class children. The education provided was from voluntary organizations, particularly religious denominations such as the Church of England National Schools. The Manchester Statistical Society in 1834 found that children of school age formed about a quarter of the total population. Of these, two-thirds received some kind of education and the remainder were untouched by educational influence (quoted in Curtis 1948: 232). Even then, we can only assume that most of these attended Sunday School rather than the more full-time elementary National Schools; at the beginning of the century about 14 per cent of working-class children attended Sunday Schools and by 1851 about 75 per cent did so (Digby and Searby 1981). The curriculum at Sunday Schools was not overly impressive, and often consisted of meaningless incantations of the catechism and prayers. Children were often made to go by their parents as a sign of respectability, although the odd outing was often looked forward to by the children (Roberts 1971: 174).

Ragged Schools were also established by evangelicals for the children of the poor, partly motivated to serve as a rudimentary 'civilizing' agency for the 'street-arab' population and to serve as an antidote to delinquency (McLeish 1969: 50). Instruction was free; there were no rules for regular attendance or dress. Ragged Schools provided a range of services beyond reading and writing instruction. Early concerns in the Ragged School movement with spiritual regeneration were balanced with concerns for children's physical and material well-being. The Manchester and Salford Ragged School Union in the 1880s had 28 volunteer Visiting Officers to regulate children's attendance and physical well-being. Teachers were idealistic volunteers, usually from a nonconformist background, and some of the 'child-savers' of the Victorian period, such as Dr Barnardo, Leonard Kilbee Shaw and Mary Carpenter, had their first contact with homeless children as Ragged School teachers (Wagner 1979; Hughes 1974; Manton 1976). Such reformers viewed education as a means to 'rescue' working-class children, supported the provision of free elementary schooling, and believed in the equal potential of all children (Manton 1976: 249).

From the beginning of the nineteenth century, teaching in elementary schools was mechanical and relied on rote learning. Discipline was rigid and repressive and the curriculum restricted to reading and Bible teaching, less frequently including writing and arithmetic (Stone 1969). The method of teaching in elementary schools was almost totally 'monitorial'. The essence of this method was that the teacher did no direct teaching, but selected certain of the older pupils as 'monitors'. Monitors instructed small groups of pupils, while the teacher acted as supervisor, examiner and disciplinarian. Although improvements were made in the monitorial system during the nineteenth century, for instance with the introduction of pupil–teachers, it remained the norm until well into the Board School years after 1870.

Government grants were given to schools for each child who attended at least 140 days in the year and passed an examination in the 'three Rs' (and plain needlework for girls). The Newcastle Commission of Inquiry 1858–61, however, complained of irregular attendance and a lack of proficiency in the three Rs. From 1862, the Education Secretary Robert Lowe introduced more stringent criteria for subsidy. This was the Revised Code, known to teachers as 'Payment by Results', which was to haunt the education system for thirty years and set the parameters of debate around the 1888 Royal Commission. Robert Lowe was a Liberal, but more in tune with the Whig era of the early nineteenth century; he staunchly believed in laissez-faire and followed Darwin's conception, via Herbert Spencer, of 'the survival of the fittest'. He wanted to create a competitive educational system which could be modelled on the reformed civil service entrance examination. Lowe did not claim to be an educationalist, but was concerned with maintaining an efficient but stratified industrial society based on a class hierarchy. In 1867 he proclaimed:

> I do not think it is any part of the duty of the government to prescribe what people should learn, except in the case of the poor, where time is so limited that we must fix upon a few elementary subjects to get anything done at all ... The lower classes ought to be educated to discharge the duties cast upon them. They should

be educated that they may appreciate and defer to a higher cultivation when they meet it, and the higher classes ought to be educated in a very different manner, in order that they may exhibit to the lower classes that higher education to which, if they were shown to them, they would bow down and defer.

(quoted in Wardle 1970: 25)

The Codes were not, then, designed to create parity with middle-class education. In fact, Lowe told Parliament,

I cannot promise the House that this system will be an economical one, and I cannot promise that it will be an efficient one, but I can promise that it will either be one or the other. If it is not cheap, it shall be efficient; if it is not efficient it shall be cheap.

(quoted in Curtis 1948: 258)

Children were ranked in six 'Standards' according to age alone, from Standard 1 at age 7 to Standard 6 at age 12; and no child was to be examined twice in the same standard. Grants were given according to the Standards and attendance. The tests were on reading, writing and arithmetic (and needlework for girls); in 1867 history and geography were also introduced to the Codes. Grants could be withheld or reduced if the inspector was not satisfied with the lighting, drainage or ventilation of the school, or if the logbook of attendance was not kept up to date. The result of introducing the Codes was enormous pressure, both on pupils, who had to complete annual examinations, and on teachers, who had to ensure these standards at any cost to maintain grants.

The education of girls was also class segregated (Purvis 1989). Before the 1870 Education Act the state of the working-class girl's schooling was similar to that of a working-class boy's, in that it comprised only reading, religious instruction and a little writing. It tended to be short, and lasted as long as they were not usefully employed. However, the elementary schooling of girls anticipated their adult domestic roles, centring on sewing and cleaning (Turnbull 1987). The needlework regulations of the Codes of 1862 reinforced the differential treatment of boys and girls. The Codes were lenient to girls in maths, expecting them not to be adapted to such thinking. As Carol Dyhouse (1981) points out, there was a strong current of opinion in mid-Victorian society that the poor were responsible for their poverty, and a great many reformers sought to change behaviour rather than conditions. The earlier scepticism of the use of schools to encourage self-help, epitomized by Samuel Smiles' comment that 'one good mother is worth a thousand schoolmasters', gave way to the belief that future mothers could be trained for motherhood, not only in schools but also through a host of organizations such as the Ladies' Visiting Society, Sanitary Associations and Health Visitors.

Through the system of education, children from all classes during the nineteenth and early twentieth centuries became 'apprentices' to citizenship, but for the duration of childhood were denied any access to such citizenship. As Joseph Melling (1991) comments, working people were admitted to citizenship on the understanding that they met the moral requirements and were not 'malingerers' or 'criminals'; so with the contemporary concerns over religion and morality an opportunity was provided in which working-class children could be instructed into being 'worthy' and 'responsible' citizens.

Feminists have recently questioned the employment 'protection' legislation of the nineteenth-century coal industry (John 1984) and the potteries (Harrison 1990). They show that the public agitation and state intervention that occurred between the 1880s and the early twentieth century represented a shift from concern with general working conditions to a sex-specific surveillance, restriction and exclusion of women from employment. Children too were identified as a social group in particular need of protection. Throughout the period under study, legislation was introduced to exclude children from employment or to establish a close surveillance on child workers through licensing and inspection.

The issues of children's employment and citizenship are closely linked, suggests T.H. Marshall's model of citizenship, where civil, political and social citizenship are dependent on the state's ability to check the inequality inherent in a capitalist system through the provision of social welfare and legal rights (Marshall 1981). Marshall's theory was largely addressed to working-class people's inclusion in a 'civil society' through the benefits of the right of representation as an autonomous legal individual, as a voter, a trade union member and welfare recipient. Children have been written out of any notion of legal representation by virtue of their subordination to adults, either their parents, their guardians or the state, similar to the way that women in the nineteenth century were not deemed autonomous individuals but were rather subordinate and seen only in conjunction with their fathers or husbands. Through liberal notions of the development and training of children to become responsible citizens through the Education Acts, boys were denied any right to determine political forces through the vote, as girls and women up to the Suffrage Act of

1918 were denied. In short, women and children were considered incapable of making responsible decisions, needing the benefit of an adult male to make decisions on their behalf. Feminists in the nineteenth century contested male definitions of their sexuality through opposition to the Contagious Diseases Acts, and fought for political suffrage and the right to employment. Children, without the benefit of organized representation for themselves, were not in a position to resist definitions of their sexuality or decisions on what kind of schooling – if any – they should receive, and became subjects of determined efforts to 'protect' them from the danger, exploitation and unpleasantness of employment and an independent life on the streets. Legislation was passed throughout the nineteenth century to protect children by clearing them from the public realm of the factory, workshop, theatre, mine or street, thereby increasing child dependence on both the family and/or the state. This process culminated in the 1903 Employment of Children Act, which standardized and consolidated the piecemeal legislation and bylaws of the nineteenth century.

Philippa Levine (1994) associates the issues of nineteenth century 'protective' legislation with Carol Pateman's (1989) feminist criticisms of liberal social contract theories. Pateman shows how important the ability to make labour contracts is to the continuance of the state and civil society. Levine argues that women were restricted, through protective labour legislation in the nineteenth century, to the types of work available to women as well as the hours and times of day they might work (Feurer, 1988).[9] Men derived personality and power in large part from their investment in work; women were defined in terms of their sex. This resulted in women having no stake in the labour contract, and rather than being treated as full citizens they were considered to be in need of protection. Protective legislation explicitly highlighted the different legal situation of men and women that resulted in a gendered dichotomy of political life. The public world of 'reasoned' political and economic life was conceptualized as in opposition to the subjective private world of the family, the body, the mundane and the sexual. Women's social confinement in the private sphere was not maintained by labour legislation alone: women were also alienated from independent contractual relations by legislation concerning marriage. Acts of Parliament removed women from 'unsuitable' work and systematically defined them out of political and economic participation, except in the contained and highly controlled environment of the home.

During the nineteenth century, children were excluded from particular occupations at the same time as women, often for very similar reasons,[10] in particular the portrayal by reformers of 'moral danger' to women and children, and the dangers posed by the 'corruptible' and 'degrading' surroundings of mines and factories (John 1984). Also, some occupations, such as coalface work, were considered unsuitable to the physical make-up of women and children. In addition, parliamentary and philanthropic commentators believed that the participation of married women in paid employment entailed neglect of women's responsibilities to their children and husbands, and that this neglect in turn would lead to a 'crisis' in the family and British society (Levine 1987). Not so surprisingly, the mid-Victorian exclusion of women and children from these occupations provided the opportunity for men to become the largest, and often sole, financial contributors to families, and thus able to invoke the moral bargaining power of a 'family wage' (Dyhouse 1989).

Children were not restricted only from work in mines and factories, but also from many other areas of employment, including street vending (particularly newspaper vending), workshops, farm labouring, theatrical trades and begging. The movement towards the Employment of Children Act of 1903 illustrates the exclusion of children from the public realms of work and the streets. Children working on the streets or elsewhere, supporting themselves or contributing significantly to a family's economy, threatened the middle-class ideal of the 'sacralized' child. Children were thus denied the benefits and independence of a wage, and increasing pressure was applied to attend schooling. Children became increasingly marginalized into the private realm of either the home or the school. The campaign to 'protect' children in employment was linked to their education and sexuality; educational authorities such as the Manchester School Board were prominent in the movement, and arguments were made that if children were spending their time working then this was to the detriment of their schooling. Arguments were also used by officials and campaigners concerning the sexual danger to children spending a large proportion of their time on the streets and in lodging houses.

Conclusion and children's resistances

By 1914 'street arabs', child workers, juvenile delinquents, abused children, children in moral and physical danger and uneducated children had, according to Anna Davin:

> to be rescued and given a more appropriate experience of childhood, so that they would grow up to be better parents to the next generation. The child was presented as helpless and passive. Victim

or raw material more than agent. The parents were presented as ignorant and irresponsible at best. The authorities had the right, and the duty, to impose their version of childhood and their version of education.

(Davin, 1987: 54)

My argument maintains that children, over a period of between fifty to seventy-five years, were denied access to the spaces necessary to claim citizenship in modern society. The historical outline above is extremely sketchy, and for the sake of brevity ignores significant details and complexities. The danger now arises that in outlining the process of children's marginalization from modern English society, I can reinforce current conceptions of children as passive recipients of policy changes. This would be a gross misrepresentation of children's many resistances to these processes. Even today, children are by no means passive by-standers of events but have a considerable amount of agency and play an important part in the shaping of their own lives and the lives of others. For instance, sociologists have recently come to recognize the importance of children's agency in social settings (Alderson 1993). On a personal level, we know that the children in our lives are very important players when decisions are made within our families.

Children have resisted these curbs on their public liberties at every step. The archives of child rescue organizations are littered with comments and anecdotes of 'unruly' children. The rescue agencies were always bothered by 'runaways' – that is, children who refused to remain passively in the institution.[11] The problem of 'runaways' was also something that workhouses, Industrial Schools and emigration agencies grappled with.[12] Older children resisted most effectively; consequently stringent regimes of punishment were put in place to quell such resistances from these children in reformatory centres and children's homes. If children were such passive victims as contemporary discourses portrayed them, then why have such stringent disciplinary practices?

In terms of children's sexuality, despite the weight of historically unprecedented discourses by politicians, lawyers, doctors, educators, psychiatrists and a host of other 'experts', a great number of children still remain sexually active. However, given the starvation of advice and information about sexual matters given to children, young people are unable to act 'responsibly' and make informed decisions. This may lead children to experience problems in handling emotional relationships (Jackson 1982) and arguably contributes to 'school-age pregnancies' (Schofield 1994) and facilitates the transmission of sexually transmitted diseases.

The introduction of compulsory education was also keenly resisted by young people, leading to two school strikes in Manchester in 1898 and 1911, causing major disruption in the city centre (Humphries 1981). Children's truancy and absenteeism can also be interpreted as a form of resistance to the imposition of middle-class standards of education on working-class children. At the end of the nineteenth and the beginning of the twentieth centuries, elementary schools conducted a stringent discipline campaign against recalcitrant children. Drawing on the 'expert' claims of medicine, Clive Riviere, Physician to the East London Children's Hospital, devised a graded form of punishment for schools in which the measure would equal the offence:[13]

1   Expulsion where the offence comes within the law of the land.
2   Private removal where the culprit's regeneration is doubtful, and where he [sic] is a source of evil to others.
3   Birching for grave school misdemeanours.
4   Drill-sergeant for lesser misdemeanours.
5   Copper-plate exercises for minor faults.
6   Wholesome chaff to maintain class discipline.

(*The Child*, December 1911: 218)

The temptation is to displace children's agency and to thereby conform to those very representations which exclude children from citizenship. Acceptance of children's individual agency is important, as it enables representations of children as independent, autonomous and responsible beings. Autonomy and responsibility, as opposed to innocence, passivity, irresponsibility and unworthiness, are prerequisites to participate in the citizenship of civil society and for children to have power over their own bodies. Thus, children have been able to identify spaces for agency, resistance and contestation. Accepting this is crucial for those today seeking to promote children's rights.

The dangers posed to a child's 'childhood' were a major contributory factor in the exclusion of children from the public sphere of the street and the workplace. Childhood was constructed as something precious, fragile, in need of something to protect from the corrupt outside world. Exclusion from the autonomy which freedom of one's body gives, to work, bargain, vote, to fail, makes one dependent and captive. In this sense the view of English history is littered with Acts, campaigns, discussions, surveys, studies and actions which act *on behalf of* children, not *to enable* children.

Notes

1 Ragged Schools also provided the experience for the more famous child-savers of the nineteenth century such as Mary Carpenter, Thomas Barnardo, James Quarrier and Leonard Shaw and Robert B. Taylor of the Refuges.

2 The Manchester Refuges were by far the largest child-rescue organization in Manchester between 1870 and 1914. For fuller discussion, see Cockburn (1995).

3 The Wood Street Methodist was a comparatively large evangelizing mission based in the Deansgate district of Manchester. Wood Street had a 'radical' reputation for 'indiscriminate alms-giving', earning the wrath of local established charities (Kidd 1985).

4 Titles included *From Dark to Light* (1881), *Driven From Home* (1882), *Street Children Sought and Found* (1883), *Below the Surface or Down in the Slums* (1885), *Delving and Diving* (1885).

5 Alsop also wrote some of the 'Manchester Tracts', published by John Heywood. Included in these were *Lombard Street and How We Got There* and *A Cry for Help in the Slum*, which, although not as high selling, produced ample publicity for the Wood Street Mission's work and vivid descriptions of the life of the slums in Manchester.

6 In the same debate on 'Incorrigible Children', recounted in NAPSS 1884: 224–36, a Thomas E. Powell, who described himself as 'the representative of several working-class societies in London', argued for the need for an improvement in homes and surroundings, claiming that if this was achieved then the need for Industrial Schools and reformatories would disappear. The debate also extended to the favourable effects a good environment, in the form of children's access to parks and recreation, has on behaviour. C. Mitchell, of a London reformatory school, compared the figures of the favourable environment of Huddersfield and London, noting the need for improvements both to homes and in providing open spaces.

7 In Manchester, the birth rate declined from 39 births per 1,000 in 1871 to 20 per 1,000 in 1916. The infant mortality rate in Manchester fell from 198 per 1,000 in 1871 to 105 per 1,000 in 1916 (Jenkins 1973: 102–3).

8 Children also spent an increasing amount of their time in the sphere of 'the home'. The consequences for women were very serious, as expectations of mothers increased – not only financially, to adequately feed and clothe family members without their children's financial contributions (Chinn 1988), but also emotionally, as mothers available for children in the home. These increasing expectations had immense consequences for women's role in the labour force, as they were expected to remain at home to look after their children when they were not at school. This new role for women was complex and varied immensely between classes, localities and occupations. A focus on women's roles in the home lies beyond the expectations of this paper, but is discussed by Lewis (1986) and Dyhouse (1989).

9 Although Lucy Bland (1992) points out that there were many competing strategies among contemporary feminists over the use of the law. In addition, Bland shows that feminists were also aware of the dangers of using the state and the possible slippage from protection to repression.

10 Although there is some doubt cast upon the overwhelming importance of state legislation in shaping the employment of children. Increases in income, the dwindling importance of long-term apprenticeships, and improvements in technology formulated the declining importance of child labour, rather than top-down legislative controls (Nardelli 1980; Childs 1990).

11 *Manchester Boys' and Girls' Welfare Society Admission Book, 1870–81*, discussed in Cockburn (1995).

12 *Manchester Boys' and Girls' Welfare Society, Emigration Papers and Letters, Vol. 1, 1885–88*. See also Bean and Melville (1989).

13 Riviere was not the first to make this observation about the 'balancing' of children's natures. Indeed, such concerns with the curbing of children's innate egoistic savagery and the nurturance of their inherent goodness are discussed by those concerned with moral education. For an extensive discussion see Hugh Cunningham (1991).

References

Alderson, Priscilla (1993) *Children's Consent to Surgery*, Milton Keynes: Open University Press.

Anderson, Michael (1980) *Approaches to the History of the Western Family: 1500–1974*, London: Macmillan.

Aries, Philippe (1960) *Centuries of Childhood*, Harmondsworth: Penguin.

Bean, Philip and Melville, Joy (1989) *Lost Children of the Empire: The Untold Story of Britain's Child Migrants*, London: Unwin Hyman.

Behlmer, George (1982) *Child Abuse and Moral Reform in England, 1870–1908*, Stanford: Stanford University Press.

Bland, Lucy (1992) 'Feminist vigilantes of late Victorian England', in Carol Smart (ed.), *Regulating Womanhood: Historical Essays on Marriage, Motherhood and Sexuality*, London: Routledge.

Childs, M. (1990) *Labour's Apprentices: Working Class Lads in Late Victorian and Edwardian England*, London: Hambledon Press.

Chinn, Carl (1988) 'Was separate schooling a means of class segregation in late Victorian and Edwardian Birmingham?', *Midland History*, 8, 114–67.

Cockburn, Tom (1992) 'The sexuality, education and employment of children in nineteenth and early twentieth century England', M.Phil. thesis, University of Manchester.

——(1995) *Child Abuse and Protection: The Manchester Boys' and Girls' Refuges and the NSPCC, 1884–1894*, Manchester: University of Manchester Occasional Paper no. 42.

Coveney, Peter (1968) *The Image of Childhood*, Harmondsworth: Penguin.

Cunningham, Hugh (1987) 'Slaves or savages? Some attitudes to labouring children, 1750–1870', unpublished paper presented at Child in History Conference, Bethnal Green Museum of Childhood.

——(1991) *The Condition of the Poor: Representations of Childhood Since the Seventeenth Century*, Oxford: Blackwell.

Curtis, Stanley (1948) *History of Education in Great Britain*, London: University Tutorial Press.

Davidoff, Leonore and Hall, Catherine (1988) *Family Fortunes: Men and Women of the English Middle Class 1780–1850*, London: Hutchinson.

Davin, Anna (1987) 'Childhood and children: image and diversity', from Jane Beckett and Deborah Cherry (eds), *The Edwardian Era*, London: Phaidon Press.

Digby, A. and Sarby, P. (eds) (1981) *Children, School and Society in Nineteenth-Century England*, London: Macmillan.

Dyhouse, Carol (1981) *Girls Growing Up in Late Victorian and Edwardian England*, London: Routledge and Kegan Paul.

——(1989) *Feminism and the Family in England, 1880–1939*, Oxford: Basil Blackwell.

Feurer, R. (1988) 'The moaning of "sisterhood": the British women's movement and protective labour legislation, 1870–1900', *Victorian Studies*, 31, 209–34.

Floud, Roderick and Wachter, Kenneth (1982) 'Poverty and physical stature: evidence on the standard of living of London boys 1770–1970', *Social Science History*, 6, 19–42.

Gorham, Deborah (1982) *The Victorian Girl and the Feminine Ideal*, London: Croom Helm.

Hadley, Elaine (1990) 'Natives in a strange land: the philanthropic discourse of juvenile emigration in mid-nineteenth century England', *Victorian Studies*, 33, 7–29.

Hendrick, Harry (1990) 'Constructions and reconstructions of British childhood: an interpretive survey, 1800 to present', in Alison James and Alan Prout (eds), *Constructing and Reconstructing Childhood: Contemporary Issues in the Sociological Study of Childhood*, London: Falmer, 35–59.

Hewitt, Eric (1979) *A History of Policing in Manchester*, Manchester: E.J. Morten.

Hopkins, Eric (1994) *Childhood Transformed*, Manchester: Manchester University Press.

Hughes, Robert (1974) 'Boys' and Girls' Welfare Society 1870–1974', *Manchester Review*, 13, 14–17.

Humphries, Stephan (1981) *Hooligans or Rebels: An Oral History of Working-Class Childhood and Youth*, Oxford: Basil Blackwell.

Hurt, J.S. (1979) *Elementary Schooling and the Working Classes, 1860–1918*, London: Routledge and Kegan Paul

Jackson, Stevi (1982) *Childhood and Sexuality*, Oxford: Blackwell.

44   *Tom Cockburn*

Jamieson, L. (1986) 'Limited resources and limiting convention: working-class mothers and daughters in urban Scotland c. 1890–1924', in J. Lewis (ed.), *Labour and Love: Women's Experiences of Home and Family, 1850–1940*, Oxford: Basil Blackwell.

Jenkins, Anthony (1973) 'A study of the development of the Salford Catholic Protection and Rescue Society and the Manchester Boys' and Girls' Welfare Society from 1870 to 1960 and a comparison of their politics and practice during the period', M.A. thesis, University of Manchester.

John, Angela (1984) *By the Sweat of their Brow: Women Workers at Victorian Coal Mines*, London: Routledge and Kegan Paul.

Jordanova, Ludmilla (1989) 'Children in history: concepts of nature and society', in Geoffrey Scarre (ed.), *Children, Parents and Politics*, Cambridge: Cambridge University Press.

Kidd, Alan (1985) 'Outcast Manchester: voluntary charity, poor relief and the casual poor 1860–1905', in Alan Kidd and K.W. Roberts (eds), *City, Class and Culture: Studies of Cultural Production and Social Policy in Victorian Manchester*, Manchester: Manchester University Press, 48–73.

Levine, Philippa (1987) *Victorian Feminism 1850–1900*, London: Hutchinson.

——(1994) 'Consistent contradictions: prostitution and protective labour legislation in nineteenth-century England', *Social History*, 19, 17–35.

Lewis, Jane (1986) *Labour of Love: Women's Experiences of Home and Family, 1850–1940*, Oxford: Basil Blackwell.

McLeish, John (1969) *Evangelical Religion and Popular Education: A Modern Interpretation*, London: Methuen

Manton, Jo (1976) *Mary Carpenter and the Children of the Streets*, London: Heinemann.

Marshall, T. (1981) *The Right to Welfare and Other Essays*, London: Heinemann.

May, Margaret (1973) 'Innocence and experience: the evolution of the concept of juvenile delinquency in the mid-nineteenth century', *Victorian Studies*, 17, 7–29.

Mayhew, Henry (1985) *London Labour and the London Poor*, edited and introduced by Victor Neuburg, Harmondsworth: Penguin.

Melling, Joseph (1991) 'Industrial capitalism and the welfare of the state: the role of employers in the comparative development of welfare states. A review of recent research', *Sociology*, 25, 219–39.

Mort, Frank (1987) *Dangerous Sexualities: Medico-Moral Politics in England since 1830*, London: Routledge and Kegan Paul.

Musgrave, Peter (1968) *Society and Education in England since 1800*, London: Methuen.

NAPSS (1884) Proceedings of the National Association for the Promotion of Social Science, London.

Nardelli, Clark (1980) 'Child labor and the Factory Acts', *Journal of Economic History*, 40, 739–55.

Pateman, C. (1989) *The Disorder of Women*, Cambridge: Polity.

Pollock, Linda (1983) *Forgotten Children: Parent–Child Relations from 1500 to 1900*. Cambridge: Cambridge University Press.

Pugh, F.W. (1980) 'Childhood and youth in late nineteenth-century Manchester, with particular reference to the Boys' and Girls' Welfare Society, 1870–1900', M.Ed. thesis, University of Manchester.

Purvis, June (1989) *Hard Lessons: The Lives and Education of Working-Class Women in Nineteenth-Century England*, Oxford: Oxford University Press.

Roberts, Robert (1971) *The Classic Slum: Salford Life in the First Quarter of the Century*, Harmondsworth: Penguin.

Schofield, G. (1994) *The Youngest Mothers: The Experience of Pregnancy and Motherhood amongst Young Women of School Age*, Aldershot: Avebury.

Spender, Dale (1987) *The Education Papers: Women's Quest for Equality in Britain 1850–1912*, London: Routledge and Kegan Paul.

Stedman Jones, Gareth (1984) *Outcast London: A Study in the Relationship between Classes in Victorian Society*, Harmondsworth: Penguin.

Steedman, Carolyn (1992) 'Bodies, figures and physiology: Margaret McMillan and the late nineteenth-century remaking of working-class childhood', in Roger Cooter (ed.), *In The Name of the Child: Health and Welfare 1880–1940*, London: Routledge.

Stone, Lawrence (1969) 'Literacy and education in England, 1640–1900', *Past and Present*, 42, 69–139.

Thomas, Trefor (1985) 'Representations of the Manchester working class in fiction, 1850–1900', in Alan Kidd and K. Roberts (eds), *City, Class and Culture: Studies of Cultural Production and Social Policy in Victorian Manchester*, Manchester: Manchester University Press, 193–217.

Thompson, Flora (1945) *Lark Rise to Candleford*, Oxford: Oxford University Press.

Thompson, Paul (1975) *The Edwardians: The Remaking of British Society*, London: Weidenfeld and Nicholson.

Thompson, Thea (1981) *Edwardian Childhoods*, London: Routledge and Kegan Paul.

Turnbull, Annmarie (1987) 'Learning her womanly work: The elementary school curriculum', in Felicity Hunt (ed.), *Lessons for Life: The Schooling of Girls and Women 1850–1950*, Oxford: Basil Blackwell.

Wagner, Gillian (1979) *Barnardo*, London: Weidenfield and Nicolson.

Wardle, David (1970) *English Popular Education 1780–1975*, Cambridge: Cambridge University Press.

Weeks, Jeffrey (1977) *Coming Out: Homosexual Politics in Britain, from the Nineteenth Century to the Present*, London: Quartet Books.

Wilson, Adrian (1980) 'The infancy of the history of childhood: an appraisal of Philippe Aries', *History and Theory*, 19, 132–53.

Zelizer, Viviana (1985) *Pricing the Priceless Child: The Changing Social Value of Children*, New York: Basic Books.

3 The colonization of the poor

Daryl S. Crosskill

Introduction

This chapter argues that ideas associated with colonialism are relevant for a deconstruction of the ideologies which underpin the welfare state. The ahistoricism of the presentation of much of the current approach to welfare is, at least in part, due to the tendency to conceive of the European colonial project as a process originating in the metropole and impacting on the colonies. What is crucial to an understanding of welfare is the 'return effect' (Foucault 1990) of the colonial experience on the metropolitan centres. The 'return effect' was coined by Foucault to encompass the range of effects that the practice of colonialism has had, and continues to have, on the relationship between the former colonizing states and their own people and institutions.

It is an inevitable feature of Eurocentrism that it illuminates the supposed benefits to the colonies of the 'civilizing mission', while underestimating the profound effect on Europe of both contact with and construction of the racial 'other'.

> It should not be forgotten that colonization, with its techniques and juridical and political weapons, transported European models to other continents, but that this same colonization had a return effect on the mechanisms of power in the Occident, on the institutional apparatuses and techniques of power. There had been a whole series of colonial models that had been brought back to the Occident and that made it so that the Occident could traffic in something like a colonization, an internal colonialism.
>
> (Foucault 1990: 78)

The sense among the English that they were different not only from other Europeans, but also from peoples in the Americas and Africa, led to attempts to classify human beings in terms of race. This phenomenon only made its appearance in the languages of Western Europe at the time of the establishment of colonial empires (Smedley 1993). The theory of degeneracy that arose out of the discourse of race informed the practice of colonial governance (Stoler 1995), and was transmuted and transformed into the domestic political strategies that produced Foucault's 'internal colonialism' for the stratification and control of European populations.

This relation had a profound effect on the structure of welfare, not least in the way that welfare benefits directed to the poor and dispossessed are stigmatized, while the fiscal and employment benefits in the form of tax breaks, export incentives, tariff protection and the like which benefit the better-off are characterized as economic policies in the national interest, and are thus protected from critical scrutiny as part of the wider world of welfare (Bryson 1992). The suppressive effect of welfare discourse is a function of the political economy of internal colonialism in its construction and inscription of social identities.

The rest of this chapter illustrates the effects I have discussed here, by an examination and deconstruction of one of the most important social policy documents of recent years in Britain, the Griffiths Report, which led to major changes in the organization of welfare, through the NHS and Community Care Act, 1990.

Colonization in the Griffiths Report

In 1986 the then Secretary of State for Health, Norman Fowler, asked Sir Roy Griffiths, a captain of the retail food industry, to 'undertake an overview' of community care policy. The result, in March of 1988, was *Community Care: Agenda for Action*. The report was triggered by a central government need to respond to an earlier report of the Audit Commission, entitled *Making a Reality of Community Care* (Audit Commission 1986), which provided a 'trenchant critique' of earlier attempts to implement community care policies in England and Wales (Hunter and Judge 1988: 6).

In the main, the philosophy and recommendations of Griffiths' Report could be recognized in the subsequent White Paper, *Caring for People* (1989) and consequent community care Legislation Paper, *Caring for People* (1989) and consequent community care legislation (Pilgrim 1993: 175). It stands, therefore, as significant textual evidence of the reassertion in the policy sphere of ideologies that had, as it were, lain dormant since the recession that separated the two world wars (George and Page 1995: 15).

Centre/periphery

One of the most frequently used tropes of the Griffiths Report is a classic of the colonial bureaucrat. He writes of the centre and the periphery, of the central and the local, of the centre and the field: 'I chose first to view the position at the two extremes, of policy at the centre and consumer satisfaction in the field' (Griffiths 1988: iv, 9). And again, 'To prescribe from the centre will be to shrivel the varied pattern of local activity' (ibid.: iv, 11).

The binary notion at work here sets up a distinction and a relation in the realm of the discursive between two sets of political and social space and raises the question about the author's location in this quasi-geographical schema. Sir Roy does not specifically locate himself in the centre, but just as surely he is not to be found at the periphery, with which he is associated only through 'visits, extensive discussions and through the material sent to me' (ibid.: 4, 2.10).

While on first reading this binary logic may serve only to divide up conceptual space and establish a relationship between central government and local authority, there is some evidence in the text that the discursive logic of the author's subjectivity reproduces and is a reproduction of material boundaries. In other words, the relationship between the centre and the periphery is not a matter of physical distance, as the Westminster local authority is as geographically central as the Houses of Parliament – that is to say, not central at all but clearly located in the south-east of England. The real significance of the spatial distinction is the recognition and reinforcement of a power relationship, with all that betokens about the identities of the subjects in their respective spheres.

By failing to locate himself in either of the spatial locations identified, Sir Roy falls into the postmodernist error of the 'Cartesian subject, the Enlightenment individual, the autonomous ego of psychoanalysis' (Kirby 1996: 37).

> By denying its location in language, the Cartesian subject cuts itself off from other subjects and from change. Jessica Benjamin [1988] critiques its presumption of independence, the way it represses its inevitable relatedness to others by banishing them to preserve its omnipotence.
>
> (ibid.)

Separated from the two-dimensional spatial cartography of the centre–periphery and repressing the relationship to other subjects, the author hovers, as it were, above space panoptically surveying his chosen domain, a disembodied, transcendental, superior 'mind'. As Kirby has pointed out, whether one thinks of this 'space of the subject' as a metaphor or a reality, it has tangible effects, it orders the world, it wields power. It is, in effect, a 'functional fiction' with histori-cally specific origins:

> While we might find the first insinuations of individualism in Descartes, most critics point to the Enlightenment as the period when the model was first realised – that is put into practice and widely assumed in discourses. The realisation of the Enlightenment individual occurred in tandem with the rise of science and the expansion of imperialism.
>
> (Kirby 1996: 40)

By occupying the space of the monadic subject Sir Roy mobilizes a political technology that constructs the space deemed to be peripheral as a foreign country to be surveyed, to be mapped out and subdued. It is no coincidence that so much of what he has set himself to do is concerned with the demarcation of boundaries in terms of responsibil-ities and accountabilities. He goes so far as to describe his recommendations as 'the first stages in a flow chart' which is, after all, nothing more than an administrative map.

By removing himself from the terrain that he is describing, the author externalizes and objectifies the lives of the subjects who inhabit that which he surveys, which is an essential step in establishing control over them. The political technology referred to here is akin to that practised in the process of colonization, in that as a very condition of its mobilization the relations between the surveyor and the surveyed are hierarchical and the teleology of the encounter is from surveyor to surveyed, but not back again. The psychic separation of the subject from the domain to be mastered is so complete that a return effect of the encounter is unthinkable.

By claiming the 'territory' of community care, Sir Roy justifies his definition and re-ordering of vast areas of the social landscape on the basis of his own rationalizations, thus evacuating the subjectivities of the people who inhabit that landscape and rendering them mute. He assures the reader that he has 'learned the views of consumers and front line providers of community care' (Griffiths 1988: 4, 2.10) but we are left none the wiser as to what those views may be. His reference to them serves only to shore up the architecture of the space he occupies and enhance his credentials as an organizer of the social world. By

naming as consumers adults who are 'mentally ill, mentally handicapped, elderly or physically disabled and similar groups' (ibid.: 1, 1.1),
Sir Roy seeks to reconstruct the basis on which services may be
accessed by reconstructing the identity of those seeking such access
without allowing for the possibility that he himself may be or become
old, ill or disabled.

> Many social theorists, including Weber and Habermas, have
> argued that one of the characteristic features of modernism and
> the period since the Enlightenment is the increasing development
> of instrumental rationality as a form of being in the world ...
> Above all, it involves the fantasy of the reasonable individual in
> perfect control of their behaviour – cognitive omniscience
> replacing ambivalence and mixed motives.
>
> (Wetherell and Potter 1992: 180)

Discipline

This omniscience is the moral justification of the text. Without it,
there is no reason why anyone should pay any more attention to the
thoughts of Roy Griffiths than to the thoughts of a homeless person.
It is also the justification for the disciplinary regime that is at the
heart of the recommendations in the Report. Instrumental rationality
clothes itself in the garments of objectivity and fact. A fact is not a
self-evident truth but a construction of reality that serves a particular
purpose. Referring to reports by the Audit Commission and the
House of Commons Social Services Committee, Sir Roy informs us
that these documents 'contain the essential facts upon which this
review is based'. He makes further reference to 'a formidably volumi-
nous body of other literature'. As Said has taught us, this accretion of
textual material is the representation of a reality and not that reality
itself.

> A text purporting to contain knowledge about something actual
> ... is not easily dismissed. Expertise is attributed to it. The
> authority of academics, institutions, and governments can accrue
> to it, surrounding it with still greater prestige than its practical
> successes warrant. Most important, such texts can create not only
> knowledge but also the very reality they appear to describe. In
> time such knowledge and reality produce a tradition, or what
> Michel Foucault calls a discourse, whose material presence or

weight, not the originality of a given author, is really responsible for the texts produced out of it.

(Said 1978: 94)

The Griffiths Report is thus a startling example of how Said's concept of orientalism as the codification and production of knowledge about areas of the world under colonial control has its 'return effect' on the codification and production of knowledge about the metropolitan poor; the 'native' within rather than the native without. As indicated above, these 'facts', this 'objectivity', (re)produce not merely conceptual categories but concrete differences between those who formulate such knowledge/power and those about whom it is formulated. We are confronted, not merely with an individual's views about how community care should be organized, but with a technology of power: 'my work is essentially geared to ensuring that the machinery and resources exist to implement such policies as are determined' (Griffiths 1988: iii, 6).

This power is justified as being in pursuit of the 'optimal quality of life' and therefore the regulatory mechanisms necessary for the successful implementation of the apparatus become a technical necessity. By reconstructing the identity of those in need of state-sponsored welfare as consumers, the individual reality of people's lives is subjugated to the politics of the norm. Although Griffiths claims that services should be structured on the basis of individual care needs, his proposals are in fact built around normative constructions of age and infirmity (ibid.: 3, 2.3).

It is precisely such regulatory and corrective mechanisms that Griffiths proposes. His view is that 'at present care is not being delivered effectively' (ibid.: iv, 12) and that this represents a technical failure of the system rather than a struggle for the meaning of community, or rights of access, or resistance to forms of social control. Indeed, the community as the site of any kind of strife is invisible. For Griffiths it is a question of discipline, the kind of discipline that one encounters in the market. The effects of the disciplinary regime and its 'micro-technologies' of power are the production of human beings who are 'useful', 'docile' and attuned to the administratively rational operation of modern political, economic and social orders.' (O'Brien and Penna 1998: 116). All the elements of the disciplinary society outlined in Foucault's *Discipline and Punish* (1977) are to be found in the report.

Surveillance

Central to the view of the failure of the community care system was the perverse incentive experienced by social services to assign people to residential care because the cost would be met by the social security budget. This meant that there was no pressure to examine the circumstances of the individual to determine whether the residential option was in the individual's best interest. Griffiths therefore proposes that local authorities should be charged with the responsibility to 'identify and assess individuals' needs' (Griffiths 1988: 1, 1.3.1), identify 'actual and potential carers' (ibid.: 5, 3.2), 'keep under review ... the individual's needs and circumstances'. He emphasizes the importance of identifying people in need as the 'first duty' in order to ensure that resources are focused on the 'individuals in greatest need' (ibid.: 6, 3.9). To make sure the point is not lost he comes back to it again to stress that local authorities must ensure that individuals in need 'be assessed (and regularly re-assessed)' (ibid.: 14, 6.4). To ensure that this is done, he recommends the explicit nomination of a care manager to an individual 'where a significant level of resources are involved' to 'oversee the assessment and re-assessment function' (ibid.: 14: 6.6).

> The power to judge, to police, to diagnose and treat, to educate and to assess and supervise constitute the disciplinary society...As the powers of judgement, assessment, supervision, and so on, become more entrenched in the maintenance of social order, so more and more people are drawn into the micro technologies.
>
> (O'Brien and Penna 1998: 117)

Training

Although the primary focus of Griffiths is the residential care of the elderly, he also recognizes the possible application of community care arrangements to other groups of people in need. He refers specifically to the 'mentally ill, mentally handicapped ... physically disabled and similar groups' (Griffiths 1988: 1, 1.1). In what sense such people constitute groups and in what sense one can group any other collection of individuals as being similar is not addressed, and probably not even understood. The individuality, the specific identity, the sheer variety of people collectivized in this manner is evacuated by this approach. Not only is diversity standardized, but also the very needs themselves are removed from the context of their production in the matrices of class, gender and race. Griffiths, however, goes further. He underwrites the

Audit Commission's proposal of the creation of a 'community carer', 'a new occupation, with appropriate training, so that one person can, as far as possible, provide whatever personal and practical assistance an individual requires' (ibid.: 2, 1.6.6).

Apart from the reservations any reasonable person might have about the conflation of need implied in this proposal, it highlights the earlier point about 'the space of the subject' occupied by the author. If one dismantles the boundary around the 'autonomous ego', is it not possible that Sir Roy, or a member of his family, might fall into any one of the categories he has identified? How then would he, or that family member, read the following passage, which is worth quoting in full?

> There may in fact be a tendency to over elaborate, both as to the professional input and the training required. Many of the needs of elderly and disabled people are for help of a practical nature (getting dressed, shopping, cleaning). There is need for a new multi-purpose auxiliary force to be given limited training and to give help of a practical nature in the field of community care. There is little likelihood that the professions will be available in the numbers required to cover all aspects of community care, but more importantly it is a waste of resources to be leaving this type of practical work to them. Certainly major experiments should be initiated and should involve not only mature adults, but also particularly school leavers, YTS etc. To some extent this is already being tried with an extension of the role of home helps in certain authorities.
>
> (Griffiths 1988: ix, 35)

So community care, at the level of direct contact with the 'consumer', is a low-grade activity befitting a 16-year-old, and training should reflect this. For training is a critical means by which the political demands and claims of both workers and clients are disciplined and marginalized. The people who are in direct contact with the users of services in some sense share their status. Those occupying a professional status, on the other hand, must not get their hands dirty. Their training, both on the job and at qualifying level, must equip them for their increasingly disciplinary role. Added emphasis must be given to the management function to enable them to 'buy in' services, to design 'successful management accounting systems and the effective use of information produced by them', to manage and support the new community carer function, to manage the transfer of skills to informal carers, and to understand the 'contribution of other professions'.

The focus of the application of training in these recommendations is to enhance the degree of management control over staff working directly with 'consumers' and over the systems that determine who gets access to what forms of care.

> In the UK at least, these reforms seem to have been dominated by two trends – an opening up to market forces, and a rapid growth in managerial strata geared to ideas of close management control as the route to efficiency (Cutler and Waine 1993). Hayekian influence may be found in the former aspect, but hardly in the latter, whose intellectual provenance remains highly obscure.
>
> (George and Page 1995: 26)

The difficulty George and Page have in finding an intellectual authority to legitimate managerialism is perhaps understandable when one considers that the pervasiveness of this technique within the public services owes more to the *practice* than the ideology of domination. The subject peoples of empire have long been familiar with the experience of having every aspect of their lives penetrated by the micro technologies of colonialism. The way has been cleared for the 'return effect' of this technology, in the breakdown of the post-1945 consensus around the pursuit of equality and the resurgence of the ideas of Hayek and Friedman based on the concept of liberty.

In order to justify this devolution of central imperial authority, the local settler administration must demonstrate their ability to manage the technology at the micro-level.

Ranking

The central contention here is that the four priority groups identified by Griffiths ('mentally ill, mentally handicapped, elderly or physically disabled') constitute the internal colony of the domestic political empire. They occupy the periphery, deprived of political, social and economic rights and entitlements. The authorities charged with the responsibility of policing the border and occupying the territory of this colony of need have long been in a state of confusion and conflict exacerbated by funding regimes, professional rivalries and central government's expansionary tendencies. Sir Roy's proposal is that community care, the euphemism for this regime of colonization, should be placed unequivocally under the aegis of local authorities' social services departments.

To secure this domination a number of adjustments are required. First of all, it is necessary to separate the responsibilities of social services from regional and district health authorities. Health services are available to the population at large without fear of stigmatization as 'natives' – that is to say, those in receipt of social services. This distinction is to be reinforced by requiring the medical needs of the natives to be mediated through and authorized by social services. If community nursing services are required then it is the responsibility of social services to arrange that provision. The contract between family practitioner committees and general medical practitioners should be amended to ensure that GPs 'should inform the social services authority of possible community care needs of any patients registered' (Griffiths 1988: 15, 6.14). The contribution of regional and district health authorities to community care objectives 'should be separately identified in their plans and budgets and ring-fenced' (ibid.: 18, 6.34). Where health authorities are, reprehensibly, providing residential and other non-acute services, various solutions are possible but a 'formal transfer of financial responsibility and provision' (ibid.: 24, 7.10) must take place, and if the health service is to maintain day-to-day management responsibility for the provision then it must be made clear that it is acting an agent of the social services authority.

Having established this separation of powers, it leaves social services authorities with a clear field of action to determine who within the 'native' population is entitled to receive services and at what cost. One of the most important purposes of endowing social services with ultimate authority over the colony of need is to facilitate the separation of the deserving sheep from the undeserving goats.

> Misfortune rather than the inevitable characteristics of the labour market, is seen as the major determinant of the need for collective solutions. Need rather than right is the basis of public provisions and these are to be kept to a minimum. Where a residual approach to welfare is adopted, eligibility is targeted only to the most disadvantaged. No merit is seen in provisions that maintain people at more than subsistence level.
>
> (Bryson, 1992: 56)

A key element of the discipline that Griffiths seeks to instil in the social services concerns their deployment of priorities. It is not sufficient that the colony of need be identified in terms of its boundaries and its relationship to the metropole, it must also be stratified in terms of a hierarchy of need: 'A fundamental purpose of the proposals is to ensure that someone is in a position to apply priorities in a way that maximises the chances that those most in need will receive due care' (Griffiths 1988: 5, 3.5).

The establishment of such a hierarchy is linked to the degree of surveillance that the colonizing authority must exercise over its territory. The location of individuals within the scheme of priorities will turn on the development of 'satisfactory indicators of need' (ibid.: 17, 6.26). These indicators will be 'synthetic', correlating age, health and level of dependency, but they should also consider economic factors such as income and unemployment to separate out those who can afford to pay. The amounts of private, voluntary and informal care available in an area will also have to be calculated to determine the degree to which the state needs to be involved.

This calculus of need is an essential tool of the disciplinary regime. It is central to the demand for control: control of budgets, control over dependency, control over identity. 'Contemporary institutions and discourses – of society, economy and polity – persist through the production of specific, differentiated identities and, further, exercise techniques of calibration, classification, codification and rationalisation in that production' (O'Brien and Penna 1998: 121).

These ranking techniques are increasingly the responsibility of local management as the state withdraws from political engagement with the most deprived sections of the community. As social work adopts the managerialist ethos to move into the spaces left by the retreating state, the division of labour between managers and front-line workers grows, and the practice of engagement with those in need of services takes on a harder edge as resources are targeted according to synthetic criteria.

Decentralization

One of the key justifications for the retreat of empire is that the presence of the state diminishes the access of private enterprise to a potential source of profit-making. The argument bears comparison with an earlier justification for the abolition of slavery (Williams 1964), namely that by transforming the slaves into wage-earning consumers entrepreneurial capitalism would benefit from the creation of new markets. So market forces are allowed access to a potential source of profit that had previously been restricted by activity of the state. This access is, however, not untrammelled access. Nothing must be allowed to undermine the colonizing authority of social services, so private enterprise may only operate as agents of the colonial power to which is reserved a residual function as provider.

The rubric under which this arrangement is to be known is 'the mixed economy' (Griffiths 1988: 5, 3.4). Social services are to become 'enabling' rather than monopolistic providers. What this means, in effect, is that the colonial authority must make every effort to facilitate provision by the 'independent sector', another clever little concept which conflates private enterprise, the voluntary and not-for-profit sectors. Where provision cannot be farmed out then the local authority continues to have a duty as provider. 'It is important that changes in the present systems for using public funds to support community care do not strengthen the potential monopoly power of the public sector and so restrict this contribution [of the private sector]' (ibid.: 7, 4,6).

This limit on 'potential monopoly power' must be understood as referring to provision, not to the authority over the conduct of community care as a regime of domination and control. Griffiths proposes a viceregal role for social services authorities which would appear to betray a private-sector businessperson's lack of understanding about how local government actually works.

> As part of the decision making process the social services authority should take account of the total resources available for the provision of care. The aim would be first, to preserve entitlements whilst putting the social services authority in a position of financial neutrality in deciding what form of care would be in the best interests of the individual and secondly to ensure that individuals are not placed in residential accommodation, when it is not in their best interests.
>
> (ibid.: vii, 26)

The suggestion that this would provide an 'acceptable framework' fails to take into account that an institution cannot be financially neutral in a situation where the decisions to be taken have financial implications for the decision-makers. While it is proposed that decisions about an individual's access to residential care should involve consultation with 'private or voluntary carers including informal carers, and health carers' (ibid.: 19, 6.40), the final authority rests with social services whose responsibility it would be to pay the balance of the costs after the financial means of the applicant had been established.

This confidence in the financial neutrality of the authority indicates the degree to which the burden of the recommendations concerns the colonization of need. Power is to be devolved from the metropolitan centre to the social services colonial authority, and adjustments in the way public funds are distributed should reflect this transfer of power, but domination and control over the colony of need is not being surrendered, merely relocated. Social services authorities, as agents of central government, are to hold the ring within which private, voluntary, and informal care are to compete to provide services. The flaw in the argument is that the authority which is invested with the responsibility for maintaining this mixed economic environment has a vested interest in the decisions taken within it and, indeed, the final say over these decisions. Here we see the compromise between the neo-liberal accounts of the efficacy of the market and the democratic accountability structures of the liberal state.

As the resources available for the maintenance of the welfare state prove ever more finite, and as the domestic private sector clamours for access to new markets within the care system, the devolution of power from centre to periphery comes charged with the authority to act as time-release lock on the unleashing of market forces. 'The onus in all cases should be on the social services authorities to show that the private sector is being fully stimulated and encouraged and that competitive tenders or other means of testing the market are being taken' (Griffiths 1988: vii, 24).

There is, however, one area in which the market needs have no fear of restraint and in which Griffiths is confident his recommendation will be embraced with open arms by local authorities: it is the area of information technology.

> The present lack of refined information systems and management accounting within any of the authorities to whom one might look centrally or locally to be responsible for community care would plunge most organisations in the private sector into a quick and merciful liquidation.
>
> (ibid.: viii, 28)

This reference is revealing in its implied criticism of both central and local government. It is also indicative of the relationship between the two and the fear of any colonial authority that its metropolitan master's promise of greater home rule is a trick that conceals the reality of greater centralized control. Griffiths insists that there is no such intention:

> The proposals face up to what may be regarded as a danger by some local authorities that there will be more central control of

community care. The control is actually intended to be a minimum
consistent with there being any national policy in this area.

(ibid.: viii, 29)

There can be no doubt that Griffiths is convinced of the necessity
for community care to be colonized by a single authority and that the
authority best equipped to perform the function is social services.
Everything he proposes strengthens that contention, and wherever
there may be doubt or dissent he faces the challenge head on.

Conclusion

This reading of Sir Roy Griffiths' seminal contribution to the organization of the welfare state, as it applies to adults in a state of
dependency, is a condensation of a more comprehensive attempt to
demonstrate that the ideology of the governing classes is the result of a
'return effect' of imperialism. Ever since Queen Elizabeth I questioned
the Spanish presumption of England's exclusion from 'Adam's will',
the English state has developed its organizational structures, ideological practices and discursive constructions of knowledge around
principles of superiority over the undefined Other. As that empire has
shrunk almost to the vanishing point in the last fifty years, the
methods of government developed to the purpose have been turned
inwards.

The suggestion is not that this inversion suddenly began in 1945,
but rather that there has been a steady growth of methods and procedures that have been highlighted and focused by the loss of empire.
The political technologies of government, honed in the crucible of
ruling an empire that was arguably the most extensive ever, saturated
deep into the social and economic fabric. The most brutal consequences of the structures of exploitation, of marginalization, of
inequality, were displaced into the cotton fields of the southern states
of the USA, the cane fields of the Caribbean and the gold mines of
southern Africa. By various means connected to the post-imperial
evolution of capital, though perhaps not to the same extent, they still
are. Decolonization, not just as an event but as a process taking place
in the former colonies, is well documented. There is less attention to
decolonization as a process taking place within the former imperial
powers. There are parallels and inversions.

The four priority groups singled out by Griffiths are structurally
excluded from employment. They are the ones most susceptible to the
technologies of domination which are articulated, as it were, indepen-

dently and constantly reproduced through every structure, strategy and process of the social body. It is the contention of Griffiths that social services should have explicit and unequivocal rights of dominion over these groups. Community care is the structure of this dominion. It is also the site on which that dominion is contested.

The texts produced under the auspices of the state represent many of the discourses that are constitutive of the degradation, marginalization and exclusion of certain groups of people that are marked on their bodies by the signs of their subjection. The codes of these discourses are to be found in the casual assumption of the power to redefine the identities of those objectified. The subtexts and pretexts of social policy are to be read in the spatial relationship between the architects of those policies and the people whose social, political, and economic rights are subject to the architects' drawings.

References

Audit Commission (1986) *Making A Reality of Community Care*, London: HMSO.

Benjamin, J. (1988) *The Bonds of Love: Psychoanalysis, Feminism and the Problem of Domination*, New York: Pantheon.

Bryson, L. (1992) *Welfare and the State*, London: Macmillan.

Cutler, T. and Waine, B. (1993) *Managing the Welfare State: The Politics of Public Sector Management*, Oxford: Berg.

Department of Health (1989) *Caring for People*, London: HMSO.

Foucault, M. (1977) *Discipline and Punish: The Birth of the Prison*, London: Penguin.

——(1990) [1976] *The History of Sexuality, Vol. 1: An Introduction*, translated by Robert Hurley, London: Penguin.

George, V. and Page, R. (1995) *Modern Thinkers on Welfare*, Hertfordshire: Prentice Hall.

Griffiths, Sir Roy (1988) *Community Care: Agenda for Action*, London: HMSO.

Hunter, D. J. and Judge, K. (1988) *Griffiths and Community Care: Meeting the Challenge*, London: The King's Fund.

Kirby, K. M. (1996) *Indifferent Boundaries: Spatial Concepts of Human Subjectivity*, London: The Guilford Press.

O'Brien, M. and Penna, S. (1998) *Theorising Welfare: Enlightenment and Modern Society*, London: Sage.

Pilgrim, D. (1993) 'Anthology: policy', in J. Bornat (ed.) *Community Care: A Reader*, London: Macmillan/Open University.

Said, E.W. (1978) *Orientalism*, London: Routledge and Kegan Paul.

Smedley, A. (1993) *Race in North America: Origin and Evolution of a Worldview*, Oxford: Westview Press.

Stoler, A.L. (1995) *Race and the Education of Desire: Foucault's History of Sexuality and the Colonial Order of Things*, London: Duke University Press.

Wetherell, M. and Potter, J. (1992) *Mapping the Language of Racism: Discourse and the Legitimation of Exploitation*, Hertfordshire: Harvester Wheatsheaf.

Williams, E. (1964) [1944] *Capitalism and Slavery*, London: André Deutsch.

4 Outsiders within

The role of welfare in the internal control of immigration

Debra Hayes

Introduction

Ideological contradictions lie at the heart of the welfare state. On the one hand, its origins lie in the need to provide a healthy and efficient working class for work and for war, and, of course, it has been welcomed by that working class as improving their lives. Attacks on that welfare, initially set up to improve the nation's ability to compete with its rivals, are legitimized now by the very same rationale. There is currently, it seems, a consensus that controls on social spending are necessary for the general good. Interestingly, a consensus existed at the turn of the century concerning the need to provide welfare, for the very same reasons (see Semmel 1960; Searle 1971). This chapter aims to show that throughout its history the provision of welfare has been exclusive and that this is, in fact, linked to its very purpose. Whether the general thrust has been to expand or contract welfare, it has always been selective, because at its heart is this idea of improving the nation. Those considered unfit, undeserving or outside the nation have consistently been excluded.

Lewis (1998a) has described how 'race' can be mapped on to nation to produce a structure for exclusion, and this chapter will outline the particular way 'race', via immigration policy, has been used to do this in relation to welfare. The role of welfare in the internal policing of immigration will be used to explore this dimension. By examining a number of areas of welfare, from education, housing and health to social security, and their role within immigration control, we can see this thread of exclusivity throughout the history of provision. The current attacks on welfare, and the particular consequences for black citizens, are located within this understanding and are, therefore, not seen as a break with the past but are very much a logical progression from it.

The chapter will also explore the role of welfare professionals within this process, both in terms of gatekeeping resources and of reinforcing a particular view of nation. Hopefully, we can also look to examples of resistance from professionals and recipients alike, to offer an alternative voice, a voice struggling to be heard among the very powerful discourses around immigration, undesirability and illegality.

Essentially, then, the current restructuring of welfare, in the face of deepening inequality, has only been possible because exclusion and division were already integral to the ideology of welfare. The current consensus around restructuring has facilitated the kind of attacks on welfare we have witnessed over the last two decades. Yet, spending on welfare has proved difficult to bring down, for a number of reasons. Social changes, such as an ageing population and the persistence of high unemployment, have added to the bill and, in addition, the expectations of the working class and the potential for resistance have acted as brakes on this process.

> The whole history of social spending in Britain is a story of the ruling class being forced to spend more to enable it to compete, to mould the workforce in the way it wants and to offset social discontent. Which of these is uppermost varies from time to time.
>
> (Rogers 1993: 6)

These difficulties in achieving the level of cuts necessary are part and parcel of the need for ideological offensives which create the climate for attacks. The 'New Right' offensive in the 1970s and 1980s did just that, destroying any belief in comprehensive welfare, even if it had never been reality. Nevertheless, there is still caution – even now attacking welfare does not win votes. One of the solutions to this dilemma is a simple and well-tried one – target particular groups who are not popular in order to weaken acceptance of the universality of welfare. Groups which spring to mind are single parents, criminals and, of course, 'immigrants'. Creating a climate around undesirability has been central to this: 'Popular racism – which has already defined them as "illegals" and "scroungers" – gives European governments the mandate to exclude them from social provision altogether' (Fekete 1997: 11).

However, it would be wrong, as I have said, to assume that pre-Thatcher we had a benevolent social order and that the provision of welfare was inherently good for all. Indeed, universality was a myth and exclusion lay at the heart of welfare from its inception. In fact, the Poor Law had connections with laws of settlement by making the cost of the relief the responsibility of the claimant's parish of settlement. Williams (1989: 153) shows how migration into the towns had consequences in the event of sickness, old age and unemployment, with towns having the 'power of removal' to the parish of origin in the event of a claim for relief. In practice this affected the Irish most, deterring them from making applications for relief, and making them a convenient pool of cheap labour. These images will have a resonance for those concerned about the racist effects of immigration control today. What we will see is that the centrality of nationality for claims upon welfare existed long before large-scale black migration for settlement to the UK. As shown by Williams (1989, 1996) and Cohen (1996) both the demands for immigration control and the struggle for welfare over the last century have been based on the idea of maintaining and improving 'the nation' and its stock.

In the key period at the turn of the last century, a panic about Britain's political and commercial future contributed to the emergence of a new set of ideas under the banner of 'National Efficiency'. Among other things, this included a concern with the health of the nation, a growing acceptance of 'social Darwinism' and open attacks upon both foreigners and the poor. 'If we are to become a healthy people, the permanent segregation of habitual criminals, paupers, drunkards, maniacs and tramps, must be deliberately undertaken' (White 1973: 120).

Leading social Darwinists like Karl Pearson, who sought solutions in discouraging the reproduction of the unfit, barring 'undesirable aliens', expatriating criminals and excluding paupers and the insane from the workhouse, heavily influenced the Fabians who were instrumental at this time in forging the early welfare state. These reformers, like the Webbs, Booth and Rowntree, were concerned with the alleged deterioration of the race. 'Britain's international dominance was seen to rest on the cultivation of the fitness of the British race, and the fostering of national unity. Welfare reform was seen as central to this' (Cohen 1996: 32).

Williams (1996) is clear, social imperialism was an attempt to subvert the increasingly vocal working class at this time, by fostering unity through nation and empire. She shows how even the trade unions, the voice of the organised working class, called for immigration control as part of the defence of jobs and welfare. So, Britain's position would only be maintained if the welfare of its own people took precedence over others considered to be inferior. This was the climate around the introduction of the first immigration control, the Aliens Act, in 1905. In the period 1875–1914, as 'alien' came simply to mean 'Jew' in the popular mind, the Jew became responsible for the social problems of the time, and exaggerated claims of the numbers arriving were used to create a sense of panic. And so what may appear to be an unlikely alliance of anti-alienists, social Darwinists, Fabians, welfare reformers and eugenicists makes perfect sense: 'For the Jewish and black workers they represent the ways in which nationalism and racism, immigration and internal controls were intrinsic to the welfare state, before the main arrival of black immigrants in the late 1940s' (Williams 1989: 160). So, welfare reform already had these parameters and in practice they have influenced the full array of social provision.

Race, health and immigration control

Since the start of the twentieth century, health, ill health and disease have been central both to the demand for immigration controls and to the operation of these controls. The very first control, the Aliens Act 1905, was directed at Jewish refugees fleeing persecution in Eastern Europe. As I have said, in popular discourse the term 'alien' simply meant 'Jew'. Those who campaigned for controls repeatedly referred to Jews as dirty, unclean and likely to spread disease, and this was to become a key rationale for controls. 'Smallpox and scarlet fever have unquestioningly been introduced by aliens ... and trachoma, a contagious disease ... and favus, a disgusting and contagious disease of the skin, have been and are being introduced by these aliens' (Major Evans-Gordon, MP, in 1905, quoted in Cohen and Hayes 1998: 3).

Near-defeat in the Boer War had added to a sense of alarm about the state of the British stock, and particularly pollution by alien immigration. The theory of eugenics, popular at the time, was to influence many social reformers like the Webbs, who supported the idea of sterilizing the 'unfit'. Many of those who were concerned with the control of the 'unfit' were also in favour of immigration control. Sydney Webb felt the increasing birth rate among the 'unfit' could 'hardly result in anything but national deterioration or, as an alternative, in this country falling to the Irish or Jews' (Semmel 1960: 51).

Right from the beginning of controls in the UK, ill health and disease were to be central to the legal framework for rejecting immigrants. The 1905 Act was to set up the machinery for inspection at ports of entry which involved both immigration officers and medical inspectors. This framework has existed ever since. Early rejections under the Act indicate a sizeable minority were for health-related issues, the assumption being that age, disability or infirmity mean economic uselessness and, therefore, social costs. So, central to decision-making about the desirability or not of aliens was the question of health. Mythologies about the nature of 'other' racial groups have consistently linked the 'other' with disease (see Cohen and Hayes 1998, Hayes 1996 for a fuller discussion). In respect of Jewish refugees, at the turn of the century a particular disease – trachoma, a disease of the eye – was to become a 'Jewish' disease in the popular mind, despite considerable evidence to the contrary. A significant proportion of the early rejections on health grounds in respect of predominantly Jewish refugees, were for trachoma.

This racializing of disease has not been confined to the annals of history. In the post-war period, once again images and distortions around disease played a part in arguments for further restrictions, this time against black Commonwealth citizens. The medical establishment threw its weight behind calls for the control of black entry, repeatedly demanding restrictions:

> every immigrant should undergo a full general medical examina-
> tion, with special attention to the eyes and skin; that all
> immigrants over the age of 12 should have an X-ray examination
> of the chest; that immigrants from certain countries ... should
> have examination for stool.
>
> (BMA Report of the Working Party on the Medical Examination of
> Immigrants 1965)

To some extent, tuberculosis (TB) has achieved the same mytholog-ical significance as trachoma in terms of its place in arguments to restrict entry of specific groups, in this case Asian and African people. Immigration and not poverty have consistently been blamed for the recent increase in rates. 'Tuberculosis became a disease of immigrants, an imported disease, and amongst the many "exotic" diseases to be associated with black immigrants' (Ahmad 1993: 20).

Pulmonary tuberculosis remains at the top of the list of diseases which would normally result in refusal of entry clearance. There are, of course, other examples of the linking of particular disease with partic-ular immigrant groups, for example the existence of rickets was blamed on Asian diet and lifestyle (Rocheron 1988). However, the most vivid indicator of the continued strength of eugenic arguments has been the linking of HIV/AIDS to black people. Particularly as a sexually transmitted disease, this has played into deeply rooted notions of black men as sexually predatory and black women as promiscuous. While evidence of the virus is not, in this country at any rate, grounds for the refusal of entry, the linking of black people in the popular mind with this virus has once again brought together ideas around race, sickness and disease which contribute to the discourse around immigration and undesirability.

In terms of how this impacts upon the relationship between black people, the welfare state and immigration control, there are a number of different and interconnected dimensions. In the first place, black people by their very nature are considered unacceptable to the health of the nation. Refusal of entry on health grounds must remain a key part of immigration machinery and prospective immigrants must be put through an array of degrading tests to prove their acceptability. This includes X-rays, and DNA testing to prove children are 'genuinely' related to their parents, and has in the recent past included virginity testing. Linked to this question is the issue of social cost. Illness may 'represent a heavy financial burden, particularly in a country such as ours where the health and personal services are provided at public rather than private expense' (Yellowlees Report 1980: mt. 2.10).

Since the setting up of the NHS there have been arguments about its abuse by 'outsiders' not entitled to its provision. In the 1949 NHS Act, Bevan ensured the Minister of Health was given the power to draw up regulations imposing charges on people not 'ordinarily resident' in the UK. These were not drawn up until 1982, though there was already an informal exclusion of black people from free hospital treatment. In 1976, 185 Asian women attending the Leicester General Hospital had been asked to produce their passports (see Cohen and Hayes 1998, Gordon 1983). In 1979 the DHSS issued guidelines to London hospitals regarding restricting free hospital treatment, interestingly entitled 'Gatecrashers'.

Eventually these practices were legalized through the 1982 NHS Charges to Overseas Visitors Regulations, the basis of which is that anyone not deemed 'ordinarily resident' should be denied free hospital treatment. The evidence to date (see Cohen *et al.* 1997) is that these regulations and their updated versions do not simply affect casual visitors. The research shows hospitals now have procedures in place to weed out those not eligible, drawing yet another set of public employees in the welfare arena into internal immigration control. The last Conservative government were clear that the NHS should have a more organized role, asking it to 'find better ways of controlling access to free medical treatment ... and to improve procedures to enable providers of benefits and services to identify ineligible persons from abroad' (Michael Howard in Home Secretary's statement, 18 July 1995).

Yet again, all black people at the point of accessing welfare are being asked to account for their eligibility. One London hospital has already been reported to the Commission for Racial Equality regarding allegations of withholding treatment before being provided with proof of eligibility from Kurdish refugees (*Guardian* 21 February 1995). A Chilean refugee, Carlos Padilla, was worried about having to pay for surgery following an operation, ran away and was found dead (Fekete 1997: 14). The implications for all black people are clear: already seriously disadvantaged in terms of their experiences of ill health and access to decent health care (Ahmad 1993; Torkington 1991), further barriers are in place to deter their use of this particular form of welfare.

Education, welfare and immigration control

The inherent link we have been exploring between welfare and nation is no more clear than in the field of education. This is a major site for the maintenance and development of ideas around a 'common national interest', and a site which perhaps, more starkly than any other, has pathologized the black child as 'alien', 'other' and, by their very presence, problematic.

Schools were, of course, the sites for the development of ideas around 'assimilation' in the 1960s. At the heart of this is a fear of numbers, linking closely at that time to arguments for tighter immigration controls. In common-sense terms, the argument goes, if you keep the numbers down it is easier to assimilate those already here, so white hostility and racism are apparently kept at bay by controlling numbers. As schools bore the brunt of responsibility for assimilation, this argument became translated to concerns about their student population: 'as the proportion of immigrant children in a school or class increases the problems will become more difficult to solve and the chances of assimilation more remote' (DES circular 1965, cited in Carby 1982: 185).

These ideas, which eventually resulted in 'bussing' black pupils to avoid over-concentration in particular schools, were about appeasing white parents and constituting black pupils as the problem. Shifts towards 'integration' in the 1970s and a preoccupation with cultural diversity in education still excluded black pupils from notions of 'British' and 'nation' by focusing on cultural difference. That Ealing Education Authority were asking parents to produce passports before children were admitted on to the school register in 1974 is evidence enough of the climate at that time (Gordon and Newnham 1985: 68).

While the 1980s brought some acceptance of the black presence as permanent, this was only a shift in the nature of the 'otherness'; as Lewis explains, the immigrant in the 1960s is the foreigner; the ethnic minority in the 1980s may be 'in, but not of' (Lewis 1998a: 112).

In the context of the Thatcherite attacks on welfare in the 1980s, we saw the promotion of ideas around 'British values' and 'British culture' which were, of course, New Right speak for 'white'. 'A particular vision of "the British nation" was central to the 1988 education reforms. The national curriculum was to be the means by which the process of erosion of the British national identity might be stopped' (Lewis 1998b: 127).

Schools as sites of extreme racism and racist violence, with Burnage being the most obvious example (Burnage Report 1989), is simply another indicator that black pupils are still fighting for the right to be here. In addition, we have witnessed erosions in the right to free education in the last few years, which, as in other areas of welfare, fall harshly on those directly affected by them, but also encourage a more general climate of exclusion. These draw yet another group of workers into the internal policing of immigration, creating a framework for communication with the Immigration and Nationality Department at the Home Office, and again asking particular, predominantly black, people to account for their presence. Asylum seekers, having lost entitlement to benefits through the 1996 Asylum and Immigration Appeals Act, must now pay fees for further education like any other foreign student (see Klein 1996: 2; Hudson 1997: 121–3).

> The government's justification for this change is that it is part of the Home Office's Scrutiny on the enforcement of Immigration laws, looking to ensure that no one benefits from state provision of services who is not entitled to.
>
> (Hudson 1997: 122)

Hudson rightly expresses concerns about the need for educational institutions to provide enhanced checks on documentation. In order to facilitate this the Home Office provides local authorities with a 'help line' if they have any concerns about anyone's immigration status. The climate of suspicion which this encourages is of concern and is further evidence that black pupils remain outsiders unworthy of access to welfare.

Housing, race and welfare

In the 1980s a number of commentators were analysing the question of housing and racism. The best of these (see Bridges 1988; Ginsburg 1988/9; Jacobs 1985) placed this racism within an understanding of the origins of the welfare state and its inherent link with imperialism. In terms of housing this was to be reflected most clearly in the postwar Labour government's programme of social legislation. Initially, black people were simply invisible in the reform programme, so when they did start to arrive their needs were ignored. Although this wave of settlers from 1948 onwards theoretically had British citizenship, they were treated in practice as migrant workers and were excluded or treated unfairly when they did try to access welfare. The welfare state, as we have seen, was never intended to apply to 'outsiders', its origins firmly located in 'national efficiency', imperial expansion and the supe-riority of the 'British stock': 'municipal housing, already thoroughly permeated with Victorian values, aimed at distinguishing the "deserving" from the "undeserving" working class, quite effortlessly turned the full force of its existing oppressive machinery against the black population' (Jacobs 1985: 7).

Black people entering the country in the 1950s were abandoned to the private market, receiving the worst housing for the highest rents. In the slum clearance programmes between the 1950s and 1970s, those areas identified as 'black' failed to be cleared, resulting in very few black families entering the public sector at that time. As Jacobs says, black people could build council houses, but were not expected to live in them. When black families began to be admitted into council housing they waited longer, only to be offered the worst inner-city estates (Ginsburg 1988g), eventually being blamed for the problems on these estates. Allocation systems within public housing are themselves rooted in nineteenth-century notions of 'deserving' and 'undeserving', and are designed to deter and punish those who become reliant on the state. The obsession with single parents as feckless, dependant and unworthy has been particularly applied to housing, the implication being that they are queue-jumping or, at worst, having children reck-lessly simply to be allocated a house. What this points to is a particular notion of the family which is central to housing policy, and which has been used particularly against black and Irish families, defining them as irresponsibly large and therefore undeserving. It would seem these ideas are not dissimilar to those we have located among the early reformers at the turn of the twentieth century, like the Webbs, Booth and Rowntree, who were influenced by social

Darwinism and eugenics. The logic which twins poverty with immorality and irresponsibility has been remarkably hardy across time and space. Housing projects at the turn of the century, like those of the Peabody Trust and Octavia Hill, had very stringent entrance quali-fications, admitting only 'the well to do, the teetotal, the clean and the deferential' (Smith 1979: 226).

Failure to provide housing for larger families amounts to nothing less than population control through state provision, a theme not unfa-miliar when we review black people's experiences of welfare.

Within this context, then, it is hardly surprising we have seen within housing departments a highly developed system to ensure that only those entitled gain access to state housing. The often quoted 1988 Appeal Court ruling regarding Tower Hamlets Housing Department illustrates the depth of this discourse around race and welfare. The Department had refused to accommodate two Bangladeshi families, although they had been resident since 1973, on the grounds that they were 'intentionally homeless' because they had originally left homes in Bangladesh. Within weeks the council had evicted numerous Bangladeshi families from bed and breakfast accommodation on this basis. Housing has been one of the first welfare arenas to demand sight of passports before allocation, signalling clearly to black applicants their need to prove their right to be here. The consequences of this for black residents are clear. For a group consistently denied access to decent state housing, denied equal entry to owner-occupation, forced on to the worst of the private sector and already disproportionately facing homeless-ness, whether you are a citizen or not your position as an outsider is clear.

Immigration law allows rights of entry to be denied to families whose sponsors in this country cannot prove they can support them without 'recourse to public funds'. Any application under the Homeless Persons Act is deemed to be accessing public funds, so will lead to a refusal. The linking of public funds with immigration eligi-bility, and indeed the accessing of public funds as grounds for deportation, is as old as immigration control itself, indicating the centrality of race to the question of national welfare. Some of these arguments have surfaced more recently over the rights of homeless asylum seekers. Since the 1996 Asylum and Immigration Act, asylum seekers are excluded from social housing in the UK. Like Austria, where asylum seekers have no rights to social housing, Italy, where access to state housing is limited largely to nationals, and the Netherlands, where the 'Coupling Law' requires any call on the welfare state to be contingent on residency status (see Fekete 1997: 13–15), we have now created a climate of hostility towards the most vulnerable. As Webber comments, 'By whipping up indignation and hatred against asylum seekers, whilst simultaneously kicking them out of the most basic of welfare provision, the government is providing racists with both the motive and opportunity for yet more murderous attacks' (Webber 1996: 84).

Again, one of the consequences of this recent legislation is the strengthening of the communication between the Home Office and local authorities. A 1993 Court of Appeal decision regarding Tower Hamlets Housing held that councils have a duty to inform the Home Office where there are questions about someone's immigration status, and confirmed their responsibilities to check status before allocating provision (Shutter 1995: 176). Housing workers must routinely ask questions about immigration status and make sense of the answers. The potential for harm here has been recognized by some within housing: 'surely what these provisions aim to do is to single out a certain group of people, who are by definition identified by their nationality, and to allow them to be provided with an inferior form of welfare provision' (Lumley 1993: 40).

Once again we have a group of workers who are expected to identify unworthy applicants and who should internally police 'immigrants'.

Other benefits and immigration control

We have seen that right from the early immigration controls the question of access to public funds has been central. By their very nature 'aliens' or 'immigrants' do not deserve access to any benefits offered to citizens and therefore, if they get in at all, mechanisms must be in place to ensure this does not happen. In the case of the 1905 Aliens Act, being found to be 'in receipt of parochial relief' within twelve months of entry was grounds for deportation. The early Liberal reforms included citizenship and residency requirements. The 1908 Old Age Pensions (OAP) Act and the 1911 National Insurance (NI) Act included the need to have been a British subject and a resident for twenty years in order to be entitled, excluding the wave of Jewish refugees arriving at the time, (see Cohen 1996: 35). In addition, women who married 'aliens' were no longer eligible for benefits that were contingent on nationality. The 1919 OAP Act created under the Labour government retained the citizenship requirement. When labour exchanges were set up in 1909, there was concern about aliens accessing them and discussions about how to ascertain nationality among potential users. In 1919, when 'out of work' donations were first authorized they were not extended to 'aliens'; in fact, the Ministry of Labour sent secret instructions to labour exchange managers that unemployed black seamen be kept ignorant of their right to the dona- tion (Williams 1989: 158). The 1925 Widows, Orphans and Old Age Contributory Pensions Act had a residential qualification. This thread runs right through the benefit system up to present day. Gordon and Newnham (1985: 23) noted in the 1980s the A code to Department of Health and Social Security (DHSS) staff, 'Any claimant who appears to have come from abroad should be asked about the circumstances of his admission and any condition imposed by the immigration authori- ties at the time of entry or afterwards. The passport should be examined.'

This research showed the practice of requesting passports by DHSS staff was widespread, and there was considerable misinterpretation of information by those staff, who are clearly not immigration experts. Gordon showed it was predominantly black claimants who were asked to produce passports, even though the majority of black claimants had not come to this country recently and the majority were born here. Gordon's work was crucial in the 1980s in noting the shift to the internal policing of immigration. 'What developed during this period was a system in which discrete and separate agencies of the state were advised or encouraged to play a part in the enforcement of immigra- tion controls' (Gordon and Newnham 1985: 70).

In analysing the low take-up of benefits among black people in the 1980s, Stephenson (1989: 155) is clear that seeing the Department of Social Security (DSS) as an arm of the immigration authorities is one of the key explanations. Since this time the internal policing of access to the benefit system has strengthened even beyond Gordon's recogni- tion in the 1980s. As increased external control has all but stopped black entry into the country for settlement, the internal mechanisms have tightened further, drawing in more and more benefits and increasing the efficiency of the agencies involved to spot the 'fraud- sters'. As I showed earlier, the definition of 'public funds' includes housing, but also now income support, family credit, council tax benefit and housing benefit, among others (Shutter 1995: 162). The 'habitual residence test' in the UK means that those social security claimants who cannot prove the UK is their 'centre of interest' are denied benefits (Fekete 1997: 16) and, as we have seen, the 1996 Asylum Act removes all benefits from asylum seekers who applied after arrival or have been rejected, amounting currently to 13,000 people, including 2,000 children. There are long-standing links between the Home Office and the DSS, and established procedures for reporting claims. The DSS tells the Home Office about claims from people it believes may be 'persons from abroad', the links being most sophisticated in the case of income support. The effect of these checks, of course, is to discourage claims from people who have every right to claim but may be worried about their status. Community groups and political organizations have campaigned consistently around these issues.

Conclusions

What we have seen, then, is that there is an inherent link between welfare and nation which has existed since the inception of the welfare state and which has resulted in exclusion throughout its existence. Excluded groups include the Jews and the Irish and, in more recent history, black people. The ever more sophisticated mechanisms put in place to root out the ineligible, of course, have serious consequences for black people attempting to access welfare. The effects, though, are far more wide-reaching. Not only do they discourage claims from a section of the population and leave precisely those most in need with poorer provision; put in place degrading, bureaucratic and expensive machinery to save very little in the way of public money; place public sector workers in a highly dubious relationship with the state; but also they hammer home notions of illegality, undesirability and unworthiness which can be turned with similar ferocity on to single parents, gays and lesbians, criminals, the homeless, young people, old people, disabled people – indeed, anyone who does not fit the model of deserving poor.

> This, then, is the shape of welfare to come. For the conditions attached to benefits shift the concept of welfare...from concern to coercion, from rights to duties. And this in turn, shifts the balance in the state apparatus from welfare to authoritarianism.
>
> (Fekete 1997: 16)

The consensus I noted at the start of this chapter around the inevitable limits on universality means, in practice, some battles are harder to fight than others. Battles around the rights of asylum seekers or anti-deportation campaigns may not be at the centre of working-class struggle in late twentieth century Britain, but there is an ongoing history of challenge which involves both black and white workers. Large trade unions like Unison, who represent thousands of the kind of public sector workers I have been referring to in this chapter, have opposed deportations as well as internal immigration controls. Each time an individual, a community or a workplace becomes involved in this, it represents a crucial stand in sustaining a challenge to those notions of 'us' and 'our' identified here as underpinning welfare. In so doing this contributes to the wider fight over welfare, which ultimately benefits the myriad other groups currently outlawed as unworthy of provision.

References

Ahmad, W.I.U. (1993) *Race and Health in Contemporary Britain*, Buckingham: OU Press.

Bridges, L. (1988) 'Racism and the crisis in public housing', *Race and Class*, 30(4), 67–76.

Burnage Report (1989) *The Report of the Macdonald Inquiry into Racism and Racial Violence in Manchester Schools*, London: Longsight Press.

Carby, H. (1982) 'Schooling in Babylon', in University of Birmingham Centre for Contemporary Cultural Studies, *The Empire Strikes Back: Race and Racism in 70s Britain*, London: Hutchinson.

Cohen, S. (1996) 'Anti-semitism, immigration controls and the welfare state', in D. Taylor (ed.), *Critical Social Policy: A Reader*, London: Sage, 27–47.

Cohen, S. and Hayes, D. (1998) *They Make You Sick: Essays on Immigration Controls and Health*, Manchester: Manchester Metropolitan University, Department of Applied Community Studies, and Greater Manchester Immigration Aid Unit.

Cohen, S., Hayes, D., Humphries, B. and Sime, C. (1997) *Immigration Controls and Health. The Implementation of the NHS (Charges to Overseas Visitors) Regulations 1982; A Survey of NHS Trusts and General Practices in Greater Manchester and Inner London*, Manchester: Manchester Metropolitan University, Department of Applied Community Studies.

Fekete, L. (1997) *'Blackening the economy: the path to convergence'*, *Race and Class*, 39(1), 1–17.

Ginsburg, N. (1988/9) 'Institutional racism and local authority housing', *Critical Social Policy*, 8, 24(3), 4–19.

GMIAU and MMU (1996) *Health and Immigration Control Resource Pack*, Manchester: GMIAU and Manchester Metropolitan University, Department of Applied Community Studies.

Gordon, P. (1983) 'Medicine, racism and immigration control', *Critical Social Policy*, 13, 7(1), 6–20.

Gordon, P. and Newnham, A. (1985) *Passport to Benefits – Racism in Social Security*, London: CPAG and Runnymede Trust.

Guardian (1995) 'Doctor accuses hospital of racism for refusing Kurds', 21 February, 11.

Hayes, D. (1996) *Race, Health and Immigration Control*, Manchester: Manchester Metropolitan University, Department of Applied Community Studies.

Home Office Circular IMG/96 (1996) *Home Office Circular to Local Authorities in GB, Exchange of Information with the Immigration and Nationality Directorate of the Home Office*, Home Office: HMSO.

Hudson, D. (1997) 'Excluded at home, excluded in the UK', in *Adults Learning*, 8(5), 121–3.

Jacobs, S. (1985) 'Race, empire and the welfare state: council housing and racism', *Critical Social Policy*, 5, 13(1), 6–28.

Klein, R. (1996) 'Whipping away the welcome mat', in *Times Educational Supplement*, 4152 (26 January), 2–3.

Lewis, G. (ed.) (1998a) *Forming Nation, Framing Welfare*, London: Routledge.

——(1998b) 'Welfare and the construction of "race"', in E. Saraga (ed.), *Embodying the Social: Constructions of Difference*, London: Routledge, 91–138.

Lumley, R. (1993) 'The effects of the asylum and immigration appeals legislation on housing rights', *Housing Review*, 42(3), 39–40.

Rocheron, Y. (1988) 'Asian mother and baby campaign: the construction of ethnic minority health needs', *Critical Social Policy*, 22, 4–23.

Rogers, A. (1993) 'Back to the workhouse', *International Socialism*, 59, 3–36.

Saraga, E. (ed.) (1998) *Embodying the Social: Constructions of Difference*, London: Routledge.

Searle, G. (1971) *The Quest for National Efficiency*, Oxford: Blackwell.

Semmel, B. (1960) *Imperialism and Social Reform: English Social-Imperial Thought, 1895–1914*, London: Allen and Unwin.

Shutter, S. (1995) *Immigration and Nationality Law Handbook*, London: JCWI.

Smith, F.B. (1979) *The People's Health 1830–1910*, London: Croom Helm.

Stephenson, D. (1989) 'Racism, immigration and welfare benefits', *Probation Journal*, 36(4), 155–8.

Taylor, D. (ed.) (1996) *Critical Social Policy: A Reader*, London: Sage.

Torkington, N.P.K. (1991) *Black Health: A Political Issue. The Health and Race Project*, London: Catholic Association for Racial Justice and Liverpool Institute.

Webber, F. (1996) 'Asylum: the government's false alarm', *Race and Class*, 37(4), 79–84.

White, A. (1973) [1901] *Efficiency and Empire*, edited with introduction and notes by G R. Searle.

Williams, F. (1989) *Social Policy: A Critical Introduction*, Cambridge: Polity Press.

——(1996) 'Racism and the discipline of social policy: A critique of welfare theory', in D. Taylor (ed.), *Critical Social Policy: A Reader*, London: Sage, 48–76.

Yellowlees Report on the Medical Examination of Immigrants (1980), London: DHSS/HMSO.

5 Clinical psychology in a cold climate

Towards culturally appropriate services

Gill Aitken

Introduction

Since the early 1990s (mental) health service providers within the National Health Service (NHS) have been increasingly called to examine the appropriateness of referral systems and working practices with reference to Black[1] and ethnic minority groups (Chan 1995; Department of Health 1993; NHS Executive Task Force 1994a; Smaje 1995). While generalized mission statements which emphasize user-equality and commonality of experiences and outcomes irrespective of backgrounds have been given high public profile by service providers and purchasers alike, significant changes in the experiences of users and outcomes have been less visible (Rogers *et al.* 1993; Fernando 1995a). I use this chapter to explore how the profession of clinical psychology has been meeting the challenge of developing and providing more culturally appropriate and sensitive services. The discussion draws on data from a study exploring 'race'[2] and gender in referrals to and engagement in clinical psychology services (Aitken 1996a), in which I interviewed clients, referrers and clinical psychologists.[3] The chapter is divided into three main sections. The first briefly reviews the position of clinical psychology to provide a context for why issues of 'race' are relevant to the profession. In the second section, I draw on themes produced in interviews with referrers to, and providers and users of, a primary care psychology service located in a culturally diverse metropolitan city. I argue that (particularly) racialized specificities both figure, and are obscured, in the provision of services to people of Black and/or Asian origins. In the final section, drawing on the empirical material, I explore further tensions which might arise in the therapy context when professionals and clients work across racial and cultural differences, and how the tensions or the management of them can obscure the needs of Black clients. Throughout I argue that:

issues of race and culture are relevant to clinical psychology in developing services; and, issues related to power pervade our organizational and institutional structures and interpersonal therapy contexts.

Clinical psychology

In the United Kingdom, clinical psychology has developed as an applied specialist body within the broader profession and discipline of psychology. In 1968 the Division of Clinical Psychology was set up within its wider regulatory body, the British Psychological Society (BPsS). The number of qualified clinical psychologists stands at around 3,000, with the majority employed across National Health Service settings and a range of specialisms (e.g. child and adolescent, adult, older adult, people with learning disabilities, neuropsychology, primary care and forensic services). Unlike the medical profession, which has the power to prescribe medication, clinical psychologists utilize psychological theories and models to work therapeutically and/or research with people identified as having mental health needs. Behavioural, cognitive and/or psychodynamic traditions are those most commonly drawn on (Kosviner 1994; Parker *et al.* 1995).

Over the years, a number of developments within clinical psychology can be noted in the move to increase its specialist professional base, status and authority in providing mental health services.

However, while promoting its status and level of expertise/professionalism, questions about the cultural appropriateness of its methods and techniques for clients, and the role of possible emotional and other structural differences between client and therapist historically have not been pivotal to clinical psychology's concerns (Embleton Tudor and Tudor 1994). Such questions have tended to be initiated by individuals (e.g. Alladin, 1992; Holland 1989; MacCarthy 1988; Nadirshaw 1994; Sayal 1990) who often, but not only, identify as having non-dominant cultural heritages. A number of these individuals were central in the formation of a 'Race' and Culture Special Interest Group ('R' and CSIG), which at the time of writing comprises a National Executive Committee and six regional groups, with a national membership of about 150. The aims of this group, which include the need for clinical psychology to identify and acknowledge its contribution to the disadvantages that people of minority racial and cultural status experience, were formally recognized by the Division of Clinical Psychology (DCP) in 1991. The SIG has produced an Introductory Clinical Psychology 'Race' and Culture Resource Pack for Trainers ('R' and CSIG [BPsS] 1995); it had a symposium (comprising four papers) accepted for the first time at an annual BPsS Conference (1997), which together with three other papers featured in a first special issue on 'race' and culture in the *Clinical Psychology Forum* (a journal for practitioners) in 1998. During this time, the BPsS itself has issued guidelines for equal opportunities in academic and professional training covering, for example, the representation of ethnicity in psychology course content and student composition (British Psychological Society 1994). These developments, while examples of better or changing practice, also reflect the historical (and some would argue ongoing) marginalization of issues relating to race and culture within (clinical) psychology as a profession and discipline, as discussed below.

As Fernando (1995b) has clearly demonstrated, many psychological theories exclude or problematize the knowledges and experiences of Black people. Further, psychology's emphasis on individualism, autonomy and rationality as solutions to distress is unlikely to be shared or accepted by all members of contemporary multi-cultural British society. This can be noted in the mainstream mental health literature which implicitly or explicitly implicates a person's culture, race or ethnicity as causal, or adding to, the presenting distress, or reducing the effectiveness of intervention strategies. In such approaches the 'object' of concern becomes the 'maladaptive/ pathological' functioning of the individual client, her family or culture (i.e. biological and social essentialism) rather than the appropriateness of the content, process or structure of the referral, therapy or organizational encounter (see Fernando 1995c; Thomas 1995; Tamasese and Waldegrave 1994). Indeed, over the years explanations for Black people's diagnoses or why psychology has not been the 'treatment' of choice have included: a lack of psychological mindedness, reasoning ability and/or emotional capacity to experience a range of distress; propensity to somatize rather than psychologize distress; repressive or unstable family and religious cultures; lack of willingness to integrate into wider society; and language difficulties (Kareem and Littlewood 1992; Littlewood 1993; Webb-Johnson 1991; Wheeler 1994). Others argue that such explanations and categorizations reflect the power of mental health disciplines to pathologize and depoliticize Black people's resistance to forms of social control (Black Health Workers and Patients Group 1983). In such arguments, all mental health disciplines, including clinical psychology, justify existing political and economic dominance and unequal power structures which have specific implications for methods of the control and punishment of Black people in particular (see e.g. Ahmad 1993; Black Patients and Health Workers

Group 1983; Fernando 1993a, 1993b; Sayal 1990; Torkington 1991). This alternative and growing literature has played an important role in introducing, and maintaining, debates on the racialized biases of psychology and associated research and practices which are reproduced within the NHS and clinical psychology in particular (Aitken 1996b; Bhavnani and Phoenix 1994; Fernando 1995b; Mama 1995; Torkington 1991; Webb-Johnson 1991).

Providers and provision of clinical services

Providers of psychology services

Concerns about the relative absence of Black and Asian psychologists whose numbers are 'so small as to not constitute a power base at all' (Mapstone and Davey 1990: 387) are mirrored in the numbers who progress through clinical training. Research indicates that people of African-Caribbean or Asian origins have comprised between 2.3 per cent (i.e. a total of 5 in 1994, Aitken 1996c) and 4.4 per cent (between 1978 and 1984, Bender and Richardson 1990) of trainee cohorts nationally. Explanations for the under-representation of Black people have been grounded in the lack of applications from suitably qualified members of minority ethnic groups, rather than as a consequence of adverse prejudice and discrimination and structural racism which pervades education and employment systems (Bender and Richardson 1990; Bhate 1987; MacCarthy 1988; Torkington 1991). As Boyle *et al.* (1993) argued, even if a lack of relevant experience and poorer presentation skills of ethnic minority groups relative to majority groups account, in part, for their non-selection on to training courses, this could be redressed by advice and guidance being given to them at earlier stages in the selection process. There has been little discussion of possible cultural biases in selection procedures, as indicated by data provided by training courses themselves, with variations across courses in the criteria for selection as well as selectors' levels of confidence in making such judgements (see e.g. Roth and Leiper 1995) and by the reported experiences of candidates (Clare 1995).

Despite the under-representation of people of Black and/or Asian heritages across professional training courses, attempts to enhance the cultural diversity of service providers within NHS organizations are reflected in recruitment guidelines and policies which aim to target members from 'racially different backgrounds', and to be representative of the local community served (see e.g. Department of Health 1993; National Health Service Task Force 1994a). However, there is a lack of available (long-term) funding resources and a lack of practical commitment by purchasers to challenge the existing structural exclusion of Black and/or ethnic groups within institutions, other than on a possible basis of 'tokenism' (Johnson 1993; Torkington 1991; Young 1992). Further, given the historical structural exclusions in education systems, the criteria for acceptance for training and the length of training to qualify as a clinical psychologist (usually six years in higher education, in addition to a period of work experience as a psychology or research assistant), the transition of clinical psychology services from being white-dominated to 'multi-cultural' ones is likely to be a long and slow process (see also Mahtani and Marks 1994; Coleman *et al.* 1998, who reflect on their strategies to provide employment opportunities for Black workers/ psychologists at the pre-clinical psychology training stage). This was well understood by the clients and clinicians interviewed in the study, who anticipated that clients have little choice but to see a 'white' therapist.

As white professionals, working in white-dominated institutions, we may be intellectually aware of the debates about the adverse impact of structural exclusion of Black co-workers at a service provision level in relation to meeting the needs of (potential) users. Further, our Black colleagues remind us how, as soon as they are employed, all too often they are automatically assumed to be expert in and responsible for working with Black clients with costs of 'burn-out'; being further marginalized or problematized; or that as white colleagues we absolve ourselves of responsibility to address issues relating to personal and professional racism (Holland 1991, 1992; Sayal-Bennett 1991; see also Sassoon 1995; Tamasese and Waldegrave 1994). However, we may attenuate our personal and professional association with racialized practices by differentiating ourselves from the services of which we are part (Haworth 1998). We may, for instance, rationalize that there is little demand for our services from Black clients, that we work with clients as individuals or that we do not receive requests for similar racialized identifications of client and therapist. Yet, for those clients who gain or want access to our services, they may be silenced by their knowledge of the lack of such choices and/or the possible interpersonal or personal consequences of making such a request. As one psychologist in the study reflected:

PSYCHOLOGIST: Quite often [we] get requests for the gender of the therapist, female patients would prefer to see female therapists. Hypothesize that because people from particular racial background are aware that there's unlikely to be therapists of Asian or

Afro-Caribbean backgrounds. I've never actually met somebody who would say, 'I would prefer to see an Asian therapist,' but that's not to say they wouldn't prefer. Either [they've] felt uncomfortable raising that or have just felt, 'Well, there is no point because – it's unlikely that there is.'

Even when clients seem to accept (or do not draw attention to) the absence of assumed similar racialized identifications in a health professional–client encounter, it cannot be presumed that this is their preference, or indeed that such wishes for choice remain static (see, for example, Sangha 1996).

A client making such (read 'personal, subjective') requests further risks being problematized for raising the possibility of racialized practices or for questioning our professionalism (read 'objectivity'). As one reading of the next extract suggests, the use of discourses of professionalism – which privilege ways of working that separate the personal (racialized assumptions) from the professional (objectivity) – obscure racialized practices.

REFERRER: I expect the patient to accept me as I am – a doctor – not as in what I am. We can all have personal views – we have a personal culture [but] that doesn't mean that Irish should see only an Irish doctor and that Indians should see Indians, and Muslims see a Muslim person. That is not a civilized society. We're living in a multi-cultural multi-racial country now – and so nobody should be given any offence on their culture.

Given that services provision is likely to remain white-dominated in the short to medium term, another strategy involves the process of establishing or reviewing services (Fatimilehin and Coleman 1998). Discourses which incorporate concepts of consultation, collaboration and professionalism are often utilized to describe the process of identifying the needs of all (potential) users of a service. However, when rhetoric is compared with practice, the voices and views of 'providers', 'customers' and 'funders' of, and 'professional experts' on, the services are often privileged over (potential) users of the services. Users may be characteristically ignored (Sassoon and Lindow 1995) or experience the process as a one-off exercise or a marginalized project with few changes in practice (Coleman *et al.* 1998).

PSYCHOLOGIST: We tried to inform the process by accessing relevant people, [and] also what the literature was saying – documentation produced by, say, the BPsS, Government White Paper. It's very much influenced by good professional practice and experience and all the forces that operate in that situation. The very much acknowledged deficiency is that we didn't consult directly with patients or potential users of the services.

It is important to note that the general absence of (racialized) users is further noticeable in the structures set up to monitor and evaluate the performance of National Health Service and clinical psychology services. This again reflects the general structural exclusions of users from those committees and groups influential in policy-making and in controlling the funding of services (see also Hunt 1994; McIntyre 1994; Sayal-Bennet 1991; Torkington 1991). Moreover, the positioning of a sole or few representatives from minority groups as representative of all ethnic groups may obscure racialized practices and perpetuate the notion of the homogeneity of socially identified categories and their interests.

Location of psychology services

The location of clinical psychology services in primary care (i.e. GP practice-based) settings has been identified as a positive development by general practitioners and clinical psychologists, with such community-based settings associated with increased voluntary access to services by people from Black and ethnic minority groups (Mahtani and Marks 1994). This reflects a more general move away from hospital-based institutions as an attempt to normalize the experience and reduce the stigma of seeking professional help (Day and Wren 1994; Moodley 1995). However, one danger is that access to services becomes largely theorized in ways which focus on objective physical structural changes rather than, for example, institutionalized racist practices. Psychologists in the present study were aware that referral patterns to services did not reflect the demography of the specific local population served by individual practices. This pattern was seen to stand irrespective of the 'racial/ethnic/cultural' identity of the referring GP (see also Bhui *et al.* 1993; Mahtani and Marks 1994).

Although we may acknowledge the role of stigma in clients' perceptions of mental health services (Littlewood and Lipsedge 1989), the assumed clinical benefits of therapeutic interventions and the importance of educating (potential) clients to overcome this stigma often figures in professionals' accounts.

PSYCHOLOGIST: Well, clearly people do perceive a stigma still in seeing clinical psychologists … It is a big issue, I think, for still, sadly, for lots of people that we see.

REFERRER: The best aim is in the general practitioner surgeries rather than sitting in a big empire building where people don't want to go or they're too scared to go … I tell them, 'Look, I'm not sending you to the mental hospital – you come into my surgery – it's only [the] person that's in the next room'.

Yet, the personal and social impact of being referred to and accessing mental health services may be wide-ranging for clients in relation to specific or wider communities. This may be especially so if statutory agencies are understood or experienced as oppressive by members of socially identified groups as exemplified in the well-documented over-representation of involuntary admissions[4] of women and men of Black and/or Asian origins to mental health services, a greater use of physical and invasive treatments relative to their white counterparts, and the dominant adverse representations of Black people in the psychology literature (Aitken 1996b; Browne 1995; Mama 1995; Owusu-Bempah and Howitt 1994; Sashidharan and Francis 1993).

CLIENT: I mean, in our culture you just don't go, because it's white and it's middle class and it's racist.

Against such a background, the importance of time, an ongoing commitment to evaluate services for racialized practices and evidence of changing practices are vital to developing relations of trust with the communities a service is for (Holland 1995; Mahtani and Marks 1994; Mills 1996). While clinical psychology may differentiate itself from (medicalized) psychiatry, this may not be the perception or experience of users, particularly when clinical psychologists work, however uneasily, in alliance with psychiatry. Scepticism and being suspicious have been identified as necessary survival strategies for many Black people in British society (Francis 1996; Thomas 1995).

Referrals to clinical psychology

Clinical psychologists are not usually the first point of contact for people with mental health needs. General practitioners (GPs) have been identified as gatekeepers to clients' voluntary access to the various mental health professions (Goldberg and Huxley 1980, 1992), including clinical psychology. Whether a client feels empowered enough to articulate her distress may be influenced by the relationship with her GP, and the extent to which she and the professional come to a shared understanding of her presenting distress (Fisher 1991; Roter and Hall 1992). As indicated in the following extracts, these relationships are subject to professional and cultural assumptions and practices as well as resource constraints.

CLIENT: Cos [GP]s like quick appointments in and out … and being Asian I find it hard to confide as well. So if I knew [GP] was really interested I'd sit down and have it out – but [GP] hasn't got the time.

CLIENT: I come in like a pathological Black person or whatever they want to call it and sometimes I think it reinforces their racism, cos they don't know how to handle it.

PSYCHOLOGIST: Women are more likely to be given anti-depressants for mood-related difficulties. The appropriate detection of mental health difficulties in people from different ethnic backgrounds is often either under-detected in terms of things like anxiety and depression … and sometimes an over-diagnosing of psychotic-type problems. But it would be wrong to ascribe blame to – exclusively to general practice GPs, because I think all health professionals suffer the same difficulties sometimes.

REFERRER: [I can] certainly think of instances where patients of mine have seen a psychologist of one sort or other where I felt they really gained nothing. Sometimes it's difficult to tell, when someone gains nothing, whether it's because of the psychologist or because the patient is not prepared to put in the effort.

Although influences on the decision-making process may be recognized as shaped by professional and racialized assumptions and practices, these may co-exist with an emphasis on identifying objective clinical presentations, or a more individualized analysis. In part this may reflect the pressures experienced in the present day NHS, as discussed below.

Clinical psychology provision in the internal market of the NHS

Like other professions within the NHS, clinical psychology services aim to meet the needs of client users in the context of the internal market pressures of the NHS (see also Harrison and Pollitt 1994; Mama 1992). Services experience finite financial and human resources, increased demand for psychology services, and the demands of purchasers for services to demonstrate efficiency and increased accessibility (Ahmad 1993; Butler and Lowe 1994; Harrison and Pollitt 1994).

These factors, together with psychology positioning itself as a discipline and an applied profession which predominantly provides brief focused individualized solutions to distress (Fernando 1995b; Marshall 1988), contribute to the shaping and re-shaping of the very type of service which is both offered and expected. Psychologists in the present study reported a pressure to provide 'effective GP practice style consultations' (see also Day and Wren 1994). As noted elsewhere (Ridley 1995), clients disadvantaged by these administrative and therapy intervention changes include those of different 'racial' and/or 'cultural' origins to the therapist, particularly when there is a history of mistrust between services and particular social groups.

PSYCHOLOGIST: A lot of people need the time, especially people who are not of the same culture or race. It takes longer to establish an alliance definitely because there's a lot of checking in. Particularly like with language difficulties or communication difficulties. Within the therapeutic dyad there's a lot more business to get through before you can get on to therapy in a way. [It's] to do with the trust, understanding the therapeutic relations and some [clients] that I've seen have come really not expecting that it's gonna be helpful and not trusting me as a white professional.

The management of the tensions arising from the type of service we would like to provide and those which we can pragmatically offer varies, which may create professional and personal dilemmas for (individual) service providers. From all the professionals (psychologists and general practitioners) discourses of compromise and/or the use of empirical evidence emerged to justify that, in the context of limited resources, service provision can be 'good enough'.

Though good enough from a psychologist's perspective, this may be differently experienced by a client. She may feel she needs longer-term therapeutic input; be aware that others have access to such resources which the system denies her; and draw on her experiences of the adverse impact on herself of being Black in white British society.

CLIENT: It's funny, you know, every time she asks me, 'I'm going to have twelve [sessions] and is that all right?' I think, 'Well, what can I say? It's all I'm entitled to here'.

CLIENT: I still wouldn't mind having a counsellor. [Black author] has a counsellor all the time. It's like they stitch you up and put you back out in society again – you rip again, and stitch. I mean what's going on if you're doing things like that? You see being Black in an oppressive society, you see it whether you want to or not. It does hurt me that Black people are breaking up.

The question which arises is how services can develop in ways which are open to external scrutiny, achieve targets of greater efficiency and effectiveness as demanded by purchasers and/or the Department of Health and yet offer users more control and choice over the process of referral and/or therapy. In the psychology service under study, one of the systems developed was referral criteria for GP referrers in an attempt to reduce clients' non-attendance, disengagement or non-benefit from the therapy process.

The development of criteria for increasing the appropriateness of referrals by GPs paradoxically can work as systems of exclusion of people perceived not to meet such criteria. Referral criteria which draw on Westernized Eurocentric psychological therapeutic approaches may act against people who do not share these under-standings, namely people from different racial/cultural/ethnic origins (see also Fernando 1995b, 1995c). This is likely to further contribute to the filtering out of clients from the referral or therapeutic process.

PSYCHOLOGIST: By tightening up on what the services were supposed to be about – we're almost creating more hoops to jump through rather than making it more accessible. The onus is all on the clients to fit the service and not the other way round.

In the context of the present service, measures reflecting numbers accessing services, comparisons of the demographic profile of service users with that of the local population, and the ethnic breakdown of rates of failures to attend first or subsequent appointments were particularly privileged (see e.g. Department of Health 1993; NHS Task Force 1994a, 1994b).

However, when considering the position of people of different racial origins in relation to service provision, limitations with such quantitative outcome measures emerge. Lack of ethnic monitoring data in general became evident either at the interface between client and general practitioner or clinical psychologist, and is representative of many findings which draw on 'ethnic monitoring' (see e.g. Browne 1990; Wheeler 1994). The process of categorizing clients' 'racial origins', even if unintended, may contribute to 'mis-categorizations' or the production of crude categorizations leading to under-representation or over-representation of categories (Wheeler 1994) or obscure the complexities of ethnicity, race, culture (Smaje 1995). Finally, even when clients self-categorize or self-identify (shaped and re-shaped by the category choice provided on official ethnic monitoring forms) such approaches ignore the importance and dynamics of particular self-identifications to clients themselves, never mind the meanings of such identifications. The emphasis on numbers and outcomes ignores process issues. In the accounts of the clinical psychologists, they articulated concerns that such outcome measures might give rise to the construction of service delivery as being more enhanced than might be the case in practice. Clients too may be well aware of the limitations of what have been considered to be paper exercises (Booth 1988), reflecting personal and/or collective experiences of not having gained any benefit from such processes.

CLIENT: Like I just said to you before, when has white people ever wanted to look after us [or] care for our well-being? They're quite happy with us just being statistics on that bloody piece of paper or whatever.

In summary, the move for clinical psychology services to become culturally diverse as reflected by employee cultural origins will be a medium- to long-term strategy. Within the NHS, primary care services, including psychology, have been targeted as the focus to provide more equitable and accessible services. However, to date little attention has been directed towards, or change evidenced in, the process of referrals and psychological therapy which considers the influence of specificities of racialized gendered or gendered racial structural inequalities outside the provision of translated materials or translators/interpreters. The focus has been on notions of increased access as evidenced by quantification of numbers of clients seen and attending, but which continue to mask the filtering out of the referral process of clients of ethnic minority status, and keep the focus away from reflections on the appropriateness of the process and/or models of therapy.

Working with and across difference

The concept of the self as multiply positioned and holding multiple identifications has increasingly appeared in the body of literature which challenges the usefulness of broad socially constructed categories such as race (Brah 1992; Bhavnani and Phoenix 1994; Maynard 1994). Here I consider themes which are illustrative of the ways in which participants may think through and experience, in particular, race identifications in professional encounters, and which I argue have relevance for clinical psychologists (see also Aitken 1998; Aitken and Burman 1999; Leary 1997; Patel 1998).

In the interviews with the Black women clients, they moved among different representations of themselves. The differential use of terms could be read as reflecting the differential impact their identifications had on their lived experiences and the different gendered and racialized communities with which they interacted. In part their accounts were shaped by the relative visibilities of difference (e.g. accent, dress codes, language, shade of skin colour) and the evaluation by self and others of the activities (conformity and resistance) associated with these identifications. For example, one woman moved among the terms 'Black woman', 'Black', 'African', while another moved among the terms 'mixed race', 'half-caste', 'Anglo-Asian', 'English', 'Asian (woman)' and occasionally 'Black', in addition to other pejorative terms which had been imposed on them in childhood. A range of experiences and understandings of the ways in which they daily experienced intellectual, social, psychological, economic and political-enforced invisibility and/or pathologization figured in their accounts.

In the white professionals' accounts, the extent to which they reported the importance of whiteness to their daily interactions was notable in the absence of the construct whiteness (and/or a racialized identification). When such identifications were produced, these tended to be in the context of professionally working with difference, specifically in relation to Blackness, and unfamiliarity with the experiences of individuals or cultures. While the accounts produced indicated intellectual awareness of racism and the likely adverse impact on Black women's lives, that Black women might construct the women professionals as racist was noted with sadness, rather than explicitly considering the relationship between being a white woman and institutional or structural racism.

REFERRER: I'm aware of the fact that she's only with me because I am at least a woman and feminist, but I am intrinsically racist and therefore she would drop me, like in a moment, if she could find a Black doctor – which I think is rather sad.

Similarly, for some Black professionals, the ways in which racialized identities impact on the everyday lives of Black people may be minimized. This is especially when working within a framework of objective (clinical presentation) criteria as being central to equality in health care delivery, and when attempting to resist their own devalued racial status within the profession or vis-à-vis white clients (Patel 1998).

Irrespective of differences in racial and cultural heritages, across the professionals' accounts the importance of objectivity in working with clients and a separation of the personal from the professional predominated (see also Haworth 1998). This highlights how explicit reference to possible race issues may be experienced as undermining a therapist's professionalism and the neutrality of the therapy context, i.e. it will become personalized and politicized. Any allusion to difference by the therapist may be understood as necessarily positioning the 'other' as inferior or lesser in some way, thus publicly confirming our own negative prejudices and stereotyping. However, whereas differences or issues relating to race may be assumed to be particularly problematic, gender issues may be perceived as less so.

In part this may reflect the way that perceived similarities (e.g. gender) between a client's and therapist's own personal identifications may give rise to some acceptance of commonality of experience. Increased awareness of the privileges that we hold as white women professionals may exacerbate our discomfort and anxiety, so we attempt to avoid how difference is imbued with power relations. Frankenberg (1993) has described how the focus on commonality by white women works as a strategy to avoid considering the whiteness.

PSYCHOLOGIST: In training sessions ... once they get aware of the level of what's going, they feel aware of them being a white professional, being difficult and painful issues arising from the privileges we derive from our part of the institutionalized racism. Feeling that they should do something but they don't know what, like whatever they do will probably be the wrong thing. And awareness turns into guilt that then becomes paralysing.

Drawing on an 'unfamiliarity' discourse obscures issues relating to power relations and racism, and privileges 'objective' clinical criteria and the adoption of 'neutral' information seeking strategies to compensate for lack of (cultural) knowledge. We may remain unaware of the subtleties of racialized practices which emphasize 'a cultural information deficit model' (as relating to lifestyles, religion and customs) over and above the existence of, for example, racism. Further, in incorporating seemingly less controversial information into the framing of a problem we can promote the relevance of dominant psychological approaches. For example, a therapist can mediate the application of a model based on increased inter-personal and inter-cultural knowledge and therefore increased expertise and professionalism.

A focus on information-seeking on the part of the therapist also may work to emphasize notions of 'pathology' or 'deficit' on the part of the client or her family or culture. Again, this may obscure the wider social, and specific therapeutic, contexts in which a client frames her understanding, and in which she finds herself relating. Consequently, a framework of therapeutic intervention may be adopted, within which the client is held responsible for providing the solutions to overt symptomatology without any consideration of the social, economic and political factors which clients experience and understand to be interwoven in their experience of distress (Holland 1995). Subsequently, a client may choose not to disclose racialized information or may minimize its relevance since she experiences a therapist's focus as irrelevant to the issues alive for the client.

CLIENT: But she was hitting the wrong subject [relationship] – she wasn't pinpointing – I wasn't really one hundred per cent truthful with her, to be quite honest, because I thought it was a waste of time – I went back a couple of times and ... well, I didn't go.

That therapy may be understood as a context which is largely independent of either a racialized therapist or client effectively silences clients' voices and obscures the range of their experiences and needs. This has been termed 'colour blindness' (Ridley 1995) and 'colour or power evasiveness' (Frankenberg 1993).

The imposition of a therapist's ways of relating to an individual which ignore 'difference' and the possible meanings of difference becomes particularly pertinent when issues relating to racism, racialized gendered or gendered racialized identities frame a (potential) client's understanding of their distress.

CLIENT: It's not just one thing or two things, it's so many – one, being a woman – and, two, an Asian woman and of 'mixed race'. There's a lot of pressures ... from everywhere. That's what makes it really hard to cope with.

Working with clients as decontextualized individuals enables us to promote generalist psychological therapeutic models of intervention as being of potential benefit to any member of society (Day and Wren 1994), despite acknowledged Eurocentric and Westernized underpinnings. This may also be linked to the attempts by psychology to extend its professional credentials in establishing its rights to manage mental health within the internal market-place of the NHS (Parker *et al.* 1995).

One difficulty for clinical psychologists is that we are socialized into dominant models and perspectives which construct other models and frameworks as scientifically less credible with their lack of alleged objectivity and/or their overt political perspectives. It is, however, those very perspectives and models which reject the notion that theories and models are value-free, that become targeted as subjective and political. Since the concepts of objectivity and neutrality are intrinsic to the concept of 'professionalism', individual clinicians may be faced with a dilemma of how to manage the separation of the personal from the professional. By contrast, dominant psychological models and perspectives are presented as objective and universal (Clinical Psychology 'Race' and Culture Special Interest Group 1995; Ridley 1995). However, these tend to obscure the value systems which (re-) produce and (re-)enact particular forms of power relations and power structures.

PSYCHOLOGIST: [There is] always a power imbalance in a therapeutic situation because you're in some ways perceived as something of an expert ... you control the environment of the therapy. The appeal of cognitive behavioural therapy is that it is collaborative [and] allows you to look at a lot of a person's difficulties in terms of individual predisposing factors or vulnerability factors in relation to their previous experience. My experience is that all those factors are very relevant to a lot of women or men from different racial or ethnic backgrounds.

Clinical experience in which racialized issues do not emerge in therapeutic encounters can be used to confirm the validity of the approaches we adopt. For example, awareness of the possible role of a therapist's own racial identification in silencing a client may be minimized if there is seen to be an absence of referrals which are explicitly linked to (overt or extreme) racist incidents. Similarly, we may identify the specific culture of a client as particularly problematic. As 'educated' professionals and clinicians, we are likely to be aware of the adverse implications and consequences of overt racist and sexist assumptions, but attempt to minimize these structural differences within a therapy encounter, while at the same time acknowledging cultural diversity. This may frame how our clinical experience confirms themes and patterns within and across clients which draw on notions of excess or 'deficits' of characteristics relative to the ways in which we as members of dominant groups position ourselves.

Paradoxically, we may then find ourselves adopting terminology that emphasizes devaluation of certain characteristics (e.g. subservience) rather than the valuing of others (e.g. connection, respect), and as stereotypically associated with particular cultural groups.

PSYCHOLOGIST: Being honest about my experience, it's been quite different of the African-Caribbean women that I see compared to Asian women. My experience of a lot of the Asian women is women who feel quite oppressed, often are depressed, and their expectations of what I can offer are very low. I don't think I would like to use the word 'subservient' but ... I often feel ill at ease with how somebody's relating to me in terms of having expectations about authority and ways that perhaps – other professionals have interacted with them. In contrast a lot of young ... well, people whose backgrounds are Afro-Caribbean-African, are actually often quite assertive and sometimes angry and aggressive initially – expecting hostile reaction. There are, you know, this great range of exceptions.

Despite attempts to present as neutral and objective within a therapy context, there is always the likelihood of making intentional and/or unintentional culturally inappropriate or offensive assumptions, which may materialize in the ways we relate to Black women clients (see also Ridley 1995). The issue is not to deny that this will happen, but to develop an awareness and ability to deal with the consequences in ways that are of benefit to the client as opposed to protecting our own personal and professional self-images (Thomas 1995).

Unless therapists undertake such tasks, then the degree to which services may be said to be culturally sensitive and appropriate may be experienced by clients as limited (with clients downwardly revising their expectations, using symbolic or actual withdrawal from therapy through non-disclosure or failing to attend sessions (Aitken 1998)).

In this section I have argued that although aware of the social and institutional role of racism in British society, in direct (face-to-face) encounters, professionals may draw on a range of strategies to avoid uncomfortable and problematic and sensitive interpersonal issues (racism), and to avoid association with overt racist practices. However, the risks are that the needs of clients will be obscured, and we as clinicians remain unaware of how racialized assumptions inform our practice and work against those very clients with whom we are attempting to engage in a therapeutic encounter.

Conclusion

In this chapter, I have presented some examples of the challenges that face clinical psychology in developing more culturally appropriate and sensitive services. Accounts produced by referrers to, and providers and users of, clinical psychology services located in primary care settings were used to illustrate limitations of approaches which treat health and therapy encounters as independent from any social context. The challenges for clinical psychology are, I would argue, wide-ranging. As a profession, not only do we need to consider the cultural diversity of our own professional body, but also to start to identify and question our theories and models for racialized assumptions and practices across the specific and general contexts in which (mental) health professional and client interactions take place.

Notes

1   In this context the term 'Black' (and 'white') is capitalized as a political category and marker of the exploitation of Black peoples by white British peoples. It is not intended to obscure the diversity, multiplicity or dynamic aspects of people's self-identifications, or experiences.
2   The use of inverted commas for the initial use of the term 'race' is intended as a marker that the author does not subscribe to the notion that race is a biological 'fact'.
3   I thank the participants for their involvement in the original project.
4   Sectioning: involuntary referrals/compulsory admissions to acute psychiatric services as detailed under the sections of the Mental Health Act (1983). The period of compulsory detainment and the review period is dependent on the section under which a person is admitted.

References

Ahmad, W. (1993) 'Promoting equitable health and health care: a case for action', in W. Ahmad (ed.), *'Race' and Health in Contemporary Britain*, Buckingham: Open University Press, 201–14.

Aitken, G. (1996a) 'Exploring 'race' and gender in referrals to, and engagement in, clinical psychology services', unpublished thesis, held at Department of Clinical Psychology, University of Manchester.

——(1996b) 'The present absence/pathologized presence of black women in mental health services', in E. Burman, G. Aitken, P. Alldred, R. Allwood, T. Billington, B. Goldberg, C. Heenan, A. Gordo Lopez, D. Marks and S. Warner, *Psychology, Discourse, Practice: From Regulation to Resistance*, London: Taylor and Francis, Chapter 5.

——(1996c) 'Issues for clinical psychology training in relation to people of African-Caribbean and Asian origins – a preliminary study', unpublished Small Scale Research Project No. 1, held at Department of Clinical Psychology, University of Manchester.

——(1998) 'Reflections on working with and across differences: race and professional differences in clinical psychology therapy encounters', *Clinical Psychology Forum*, 118, 11–17.

Aitken, G. and Burman, E. (1999) 'Keeping and crossing professional and racialized boundaries: implications for feminist practice', to appear in Special Issue on Innovative Methods: *Psychology of Women Quarterly*, March–June 1999.

Alladin, W. (1992) 'Clinical psychology provision', in W. Ahmad (ed.), *Politics of Race and Health*, Bradford: University of Bradford Print Unit, 117–42.

Bender, M. and Richardson, A. (1990) 'The ethnic composition of clinical psychology in Britain', *The Psychologist: Bulletin of the British Psychological Society*, 6, 250–2.

Bhate, S. (1987) 'Prejudice against doctors and students from ethnic minorities', *British Medical Journal*, 294, 838.

Bhavnani, K. and Phoenix, A. (1994) 'Shifting identities shifting racisms: an introduction', *Feminism and Psychology*, 4, 5–18.

Bhui, K., Strathdee, G. and Sufraz, R. (1993) 'Asian inpatients in a district psychiatric unit: an examination of presenting features and routes into care', *International Journal of Social Psychiatry*, 39, 208–20.

Black Health Workers and Patients Group (1983) 'Psychiatry and the corporate state', *Race and Class* XXV, 249–64.

Booth, H. (1988) 'Identifying ethnic origin: the past, present and future of official data production', in A. Bhat, R. Carr Hill and S. Ohri (eds), *Britain's Black Population: A New Perspective*, Aldershot: Gower, 237–68.

Boyle, M., Baker, M., Bennett, E. and Charman, T. (1993) 'Selection for clinical psychology courses: a comparison of applicants from ethnic minority and majority groups to the University of East London', *Clinical Psychology Forum*, 56, 9–13.

Brah, A. (1992) 'Difference, diversity and differentiation', in J. Donald and A. Rattansi (eds), *'Race', Culture and Difference*, Buckingham: Open University Press/Sage, 126–48.

British Psychological Society (1994) 'Equal opportunities policy,' *The Psychologist: Bulletin of the British Psychological Society*, 6, 178.

Browne, D. (1990) *Black People, Mental Health and the Courts*, London: National Association for the Care and Resettlement of Offenders (NACRO).

—— (1995) 'Sectioning: the Black experience', in S. Fernando (ed.), *Mental Health in a Multi-Ethnic Society: A Multi-Disciplinary Handbook*, London: Routledge, 36–50.

Butler, G. and Lowe, J. (1994) 'Short-term psychotherapy', in P. Clarkson and M. Pokorny (eds), *The Handbook of Psychotherapy*, London: Routledge, 208–24.

Chan, M. (1995) 'The NHS response to minority ethnic health: improving services for Asian people with learning disabilities', paper presented at A One-Day Event for Asian Staff, University of Manchester (April).

Clare, L. (1995) 'Successful applicants for clinical training: a descriptive profile of one trainee cohort', *Clinical Psychology Forum*, 77, 31–4.

Clinical Psychology 'Race' and Culture Special Interest Group of the British Psychological Society [Division of Clinical Psychology] (1995) *Clinical Psychology 'Race' and Culture Resource Pack for Trainers*, British Psychological Society.

Coleman, P.G., Brown, R., Acton, C., Harris, A., and Saltmore, S. (1998) 'Building links with a black community: experiences in central Manchester', *Clinical Psychology Forum*, 118, 43–8.

Day, C. and Wren, B. (1994) 'Journey to the centre of primary care: primary care psychology in perspective', *Clinical Psychology Forum*, 65, 3–6.

Department of Health (1993) *Ethnicity and Health: A Guide for the NHS*, London: HMSO.

Embleton Tudor, L. and Tudor, K. (1994) 'The personal and the political: power, authority and influence in psychotherapy', in P. Clarkson and M. Pokorny (eds), *The Handbook of Psychotherapy*, London: Routledge, 384–402.

Fatimilehin, I. and Coleman, P.G. (1998) 'Appropriate services for African Caribbean families: views from one community', *Clinical Psychology Forum*, 111, 6–11.

Fernando, S. (1993a) 'Psychiatry and racism', *Changes*, 11, 46–58.

—— (1993b) 'Racial bias and schizophrenia', *Transcultural Psychiatry Society Bulletin*, 2, 9–13.

—— (1995a) 'Introduction', in S. Fernando (ed.), *Mental Health in a Multi-Ethnic Society: A Multi-Disciplinary Handbook*, London: Routledge, 1–10.

—— (1995b) 'Social realities and mental health', in S. Fernando (ed.), *Mental Health in a Multi-Ethnic Society: A Multi-Disciplinary Handbook*, London: Routledge, 11–35.

—— (1995c) 'Professional interventions: therapy and care', in S. Fernando (ed.), *Mental Health in a Multi-Ethnic Society: A Multi-Disciplinary Handbook*, London: Routledge, 36–50.

Fisher, S. (1991) 'A discourse of the social: medical talk/power talk/oppositional talk?', *Discourse and Society*, 2, 157–82.

Francis, E. (1996) 'A crisis in social care: a framework for understanding the mental health predicament facing Britain's black communities', paper presented at Working with Diversity and Differences Conference, ORT House Conference Centre, Camden: Pavilion/Avelon Associates (June).

Frankenberg, R. (1993) *The Social Construction of Whiteness: White Women, Race Matters*, London: Routledge.

Goldberg, D. and Huxley, P. (1980) *Mental Illness in the Community*, London: Tavistock.

——(1992) *Common Mental Disorders*, London: Routledge.

Harrison, S. and Pollitt, C. (1994) *Controlling Health Professionals: The Future of Work and Organization in the NHS*, Buckingham: Open University Press.

Haworth, R. (1998) 'Mental health professionals' accounts of clients who are from ethnic minorities', *Clinical Psychology Forum*, 118, 6–10.

Holland, S. (1989) 'Women and community mental health – twenty years on', *Clinical Psychology Forum*, 22, 35–7.

——(1991) 'From private symptom to public action', *Psychology and Feminism*, 1, 58–62.

——(1992) 'From social abuse to social action: a neighbourhood psychotherapy and social action project for women', in J. Ussher and P. Nicolson (eds), *Gender Issues in Clinical Psychology*, London: Routledge.

——(1995) 'Interaction in women's mental health and neighbourhood development', in S. Fernando (ed.), *Mental Health in a Multi-Ethnic Society: A Multi-Disciplinary Handbook*, London: Routledge, 36–50.

Hunt, P. (1994) *Working Across Cultures: Catering for Whose Needs: Is Change Needed?*, London: St George's Mental Health Library Conference Series.

Johnson, M. (1993) 'Equal opportunities in service development – responses to a changing population', in W. Ahmad (ed.), *'Race' and Health in Contemporary Britain*, Buckingham: Open University Press, 183–200.

Kareem, J. and Littlewood, R. (eds) (1992) *Intercultural Therapy: Themes, Interpretations and Practice*, Oxford: Blackwell Scientific Publications.

Kosviner, A. (1994) 'Psychotherapies within the NHS', in P. Clarkson and M. Pokorny (eds), *The Handbook of Psychotherapy*, London: Routledge, 286–99.

Leary, K. (1997) 'Race, self-disclosure, and "forbidden talk": race and ethnicity in contemporary clinical practice', *Psychoanalytic Quarterly*, LXVI, 163–89.

Littlewood, R. (1993) 'Ideology, camouflage or contingency? Racism in British psychiatry', *Transcultural Psychiatric Research Review*, 30, 243–90.

Littlewood, R. and Lipsedge, M. (1989) *Aliens and Alienists: Ethnic Minorities and Psychiatry* (second edition), London: Unwin Hyman.

MacCarthy, B. (1988) 'Clinical work with ethnic minorities', in F. Watts (ed.), *New Developments in Clinical Psychology*, vol. 2, London: BPS/John Wiley and Sons.

McIntyre, K. (1994) 'Time for action now: the African-Caribbean perspectives' in National Health Service Task Force (1994) 'Time for Action

Now – Regional Race Programme', Greater Manchester Seminar, Department of Health.

Mahtani, A. and Marks, L. (1994) 'Developing a primary care psychology service that is racially and culturally appropriate', *Clinical Psychology Forum*, 65, 27–31.

Mama, A. (1992) 'Black women and the British state', in P. Braham, A. Rattansi and R. Skellington (eds), *Racism and Antiracism*, London: Sage, 79–104.

——(1995) *Beyond the Masks: Race, Gender and Subjectivity*, London: Routledge.

Mapstone, E. and Davey, G. (1990) 'Foreword: On being at a disadvantage', *The Psychologist: Bulletin of the British Psychological Society*, 13, 387.

Marshall, R. (1988) 'The role of ideology in the individualization of distress', *The Psychologist: Bulletin of the British Psychological Society*, 2, 67–9.

Maynard, M. (1994) '"Race", gender and the concept of "difference" in feminist thought', in H. Afshar and M. Maynard (eds), *The Dynamics of 'Race' and Gender*, London: Taylor and Francis, 9–25.

Mills, M. (1996) 'SHANTI: an intercultural psychotherapy centre for women in the community', in K. Abel, M. Buszewicz, S. Davison, S. Johnson and E. Staples (eds), *Planning Community Mental Health Services for Women.* London: Routledge, 219–30.

Moodley, P. (1995) 'Reaching out', in S. Fernando (ed.), *Mental Health in a Multi-Ethnic Society: A Multi-Disciplinary Handbook*, London: Routledge, 120–39.

Nadirshaw, Z. (1994) 'Clinical psychology and ethnic communities', *Clinical Psychology Forum*, 69, 38–9.

National Health Service Task Force (1994a) *Black Mental Health: A Dialogue for Change*, Department of Health.

——(1994b) 'Time for Action Now – Regional Race Programme', Greater Manchester Seminar, Department of Health.

Owusu-Bempah, J. and Howitt, D. (1994) 'Racism and the psychological textbook,' *The Psychologist: Bulletin of the British Psychological Society*, 7, 163–6.

Parker, I., Georgaca, E., Harper, D., McLaughlin, T. and Stowell-Smith, M. (1995) *Deconstructing Psychopathology*, London: Sage.

Patel, M. (1998) 'Black therapists/white clients: an exploration of experiences in cross-cultural therapy', *Clinical Psychology Forum*, 118; 18–23.

Ridley, C. (1995) *Overcoming Unintentional Racism in Counseling and Therapy*, California: Sage.

Rogers, A., Pilgrim, D. and Lacey, R. (1993) *Experiencing Psychiatry: Users' Views of Services*, London: Macmillan Press Ltd/MIND.

Roter, D. and Hall, J. (1992) *Doctors Talking with Patients: Patients Talking with Doctors*, London: Auburn House.

Roth, T, and Leiper, R. (1995) 'Selecting for clinical training', *The Psychologist: Bulletin of the British Psychological Society*, 8, 25–8.

Sangha, K. (1996) 'Asian Women and Psychotherapy: Providers' and Recipients' Perspectives', unpublished MSc thesis (by research) held at Manchester Metropolitan University, Manchester.

Sashidharan, S. and Francis, E. (1993) 'Epidemiology, ethnicity and schizophrenia', in W. Ahmad (ed.), *'Race' and Health in Contemporary Britain*, Buckingham: Open University Press, 96–113.

Sassoon, M. (1995) 'Tackling marginalization, supporting survival: black workers, black users and white organizations', *Good Practices in Mental Health: Not Just Black and White*; 19, 23.

Sassoon, M. and Lindow, V. (1995) 'Consulting and empowering black mental health system users', in S. Fernando (ed.), *Mental Health in a Multi-Ethnic Society: A Multi-Disciplinary Handbook*, London: Routledge, 89–106.

Sayal, A. (1990) 'Black women and mental health', *The Psychologist: Bulletin of the British Psychological Society*, 3, 24–7.

Sayal-Bennet, A. (1991) 'Equal opportunities – empty rhetoric', *Feminism and Psychology*, 1, 74–7.

Smaje, C. (1995) 'Race and ethnicity: true colours', *Health Service Journal*, 26 January, 28–9.

Tamasese, K. and Waldegrave, C. (1994) 'The just therapy approach', *Dulwich Centre Newsletter*, 2 and 3, 55–67.

Thomas, L. (1995) 'Psychotherapy in the context of race and culture: an intercultural therapeutic approach', in S. Fernando (ed.), *Mental Health in a Multi-Ethnic Society: A Multi-Disciplinary Handbook*, London: Routledge, 172–92.

Torkington, P. (1991) *Black Health – A Political Issue: The Health and Race Project, Liverpool*, London: Catholic Association for Racial Justice/Liverpool Institute of Higher Education.

Webb-Johnson, A. (1991) *A Cry for Change: An Asian Perspective on Developing Quality Mental Health Care*, London: Confederation of Indian Organisations (UK).

Wheeler, E. (1994) 'Doing black mental health research: observations and experiences', in H. Afshar, and M. Maynard (eds), *The Dynamics of 'Race' and Gender*, London: Taylor and Francis, 41–62.

Young, K. (1992) 'Approaches to policy development', in P. Braham, A. Rattansi and R. Skeelington (eds), *Racism and Anti-Racism*, Buckingham: Open University Press, 252–69.

6 Resources for hope
Social work and social exclusion

Beth Humphries

Introduction

We live in a time when we are inextricably connected, as citizens across national boundaries through inter-country alliances, through international organizations and treaties and through globalization resulting from the spread of late twentieth-century capitalism. One of the consequences of this is that the nature of the 'caring professions', certainly in advanced industrialized countries, has changed radically, in the view of many of us, to the detriment of those whom they purport to help. As welfare professionals and educators we are also connected in ways that expose us to other cultures and beliefs which (in theory) influence and modify our views of the world. Here there is potential for an enrichment of our understandings of social need.

At the same time as we experience this connectedness and these fundamental changes, the postmodern critique – the rejection of the grand theories which purport to explain social life; the questioning of an essential universal subject; the scepticism about the transparency and certainty of language – threatens ideas of continuity, blurs boundaries, emphasizes difference and threatens to fragment categories we have regarded as clear and unambiguous: even categories such as 'men', 'women', 'ethnicity', 'heterosexuality' (Riley 1988).

In this chapter I want to explore some of the dimensions and some of the contradictions of these influences in relation to social work, in an attempt to review the position and to reach towards a conception of social work whose individual members, across countries, unknown to each other and very different from each other, might use those differences as a resource towards building values that are grounded in ideas about freedom from oppression. First, I shall outline some of the ideas I have signalled.

The politics of exclusion

I want to frame my comments for the first part of the chapter within a notion of the politics of exclusion because it is within this arena in which social work operates. Across the world, who belongs and who does not belong are preoccupations which lead to oppression and conflict.

Social exclusion has become a theme in the social policy of the European Commission (Commission of the European Communities 1992, 1993), and as a result all the member states, including Britain, have included it in their economic policies. However, there are contradictions between inclusionary aims and exclusionary outcomes. I have identified a number of dimensions to this: *absolute exclusions, inclusions experienced as exclusion*, and *inappropriate inclusions*.

Absolute exclusions

Absolute exclusion is where people are refused entry to a country through border controls. The era in which we live has been called the international 'age of migration', characterized by the globalization, acceleration, differentiation and feminization of migration patterns (Castles and Miller 1993). Migration has been expanding in terms of both its overall volume and the number of countries affected. In Western Europe, postwar immigration has embraced ex-colonial subjects, 'temporary' migrant workers from countries of the south and their families, and, increasingly, refugees and asylum seekers and so-called 'illegal' immigrants (Lister 1997: 44). But in spite of international agreements on human rights, an exclusionary stance is being taken by First World countries, including the countries of Western Europe, the USA, Canada and Australia. There are also examples of this in other parts of the world, such as Israel, where unrestricted access is given to some, and blocked completely to others.

Fortress Europe, indeed Fortress First World, while abolishing internal border controls in the name of free movement, has at the same time tightened its boundaries (Cohen and Hayes 1998). These external controls are increasingly more stringent, they restrict immigration and the numbers of refugees and asylum seekers admitted, they provide for the swift expulsion of unwanted aliens, and they sanction strict surveillance of those who are admitted. Importantly, these inclusionary and exclusionary criteria relate to ethnic and racial divisions as well as class and gender divisions (Yuval Davis 1991). More and more, the implicit image of the European is to be white, Christian and holding a Eurocentric view of the world.

Inclusions experienced as exclusion

Moving on to inclusions experienced as exclusion, one of the groups I have in mind is those who have been admitted to countries, but who are denied social and civil rights and access to citizenship. Many live on the margins of society, vulnerable to poverty and ill health. In Britain, the role of health and welfare professionals is being expanded to become part of internal controls. In other words, they are expected to check immigration status before offering a service. There has been little by way of an outcry against this as discriminatory, as an unethical activity, and as outside the proper professional function of social workers and health workers. Research carried out by Cohen *et al.* (1997) showed very little awareness or concern among health professionals. The focus of anti-discrimination among professionals, where it exists, is individualistic and narrow, where, head-down, the concern is exclusively with micro activity, allowing policies which are dehumanizing and oppressive to be placed in our hands, almost by stealth. The question 'Why?' is not asked.

This intensification of control within borders, which includes seeking proof of identification and the production of a passport, has an impact on other citizens. Sivanandan (1993) draws these wider implications:

> This racism is becoming one with a common European culture, which defines all Third World people as immigrants and refugees, and all immigrants and refugees as terrorists and drug-runners, [which] will not be able to tell a citizen from an immigrant, or an immigrant from a refugee, let alone one black from another. They all carry their passport on their faces.
>
> (Sivanandan 1993:12)

Sivanandan speaks here of those from racialized minorities within countries, who are treated as 'outsiders within'. In some countries it is impossible to tell by looks who is an insider and who is an outsider, but there are other clues as to identity. In my home country, Northern Ireland, people's names, the school they went to, the way they pronounce certain words, even whether they call their country 'Northern Ireland' or 'the North of Ireland', all signify their 'place'.

But these developments are only another evidence of the second-class treatment of minority ethnic groups, not only in Europe but also across the world. Exploitation in employment, denial of access to education and a country's wealth, discrimination, racial harassment and violence, even ethnic extermination. In Britain, those who have committed crimes may suffer what has become known as 'double punishment' (GMIAU 1998). After serving their sentence they may be deported.[1] They are, in the main, black men: the punishment is therefore not only to them, but also to their partners and families. We all know of others who are wrongly imprisoned, imprisoned without trial, imprisoned as dissidents. There are those who only comparatively recently have received the right of citizenship, such as black people in the USA, Aboriginal peoples in Australia, black South Africans. The modern world is characterized by exclusions – who does not belong, even within the boundaries of the nation-state.

There are other ways in which inclusion is experienced as exclusion. All of the problems I identified, associated with external and internal boundary controls, are mediated across class, gender and sexuality. Women as refugees, as asylum seekers and as migrant workers, are affected differently from men (Lister 1997). Gay men and lesbians are treated differently from heterosexuals in relation to immigration controls. More generally, in terms of the material conditions of women's lives, worldwide, women do more work than men, yet their labour is seen to be of less value. They receive on average about 30–40 per cent less pay than men if employed, and no pay at all for most domestic work. They hold only 10–20 per cent of managerial and administrative jobs, and are poorly represented in the ranks of power, policy and decision-making (United Nations 1991: 6).

International health statistics reflect inequalities along 'race', class and nationality lines. These relate to hazards at work; violence in the home; sexual harassment; sex, reproduction and illness and mortality; medicine and power over women (Doyal 1995). These 'inclusions experienced as exclusion' are grounded in inequality. It may take different forms, and different factors may be of over-riding political concern for different groups at different times and places, but the evidence for its material existence is irrefutable (Humphries 1998).

Internal exclusionary processes affect other groups also. Are there any countries where gay men and lesbians have the same citizenship rights as heterosexuals? In some countries they have none, in others they are restricted in terms of the age of consent, of rights to legal partnership and to bear and raise or adopt children, and in jobs and personal insurance. In informal and subtle ways they are discriminated against in jobs, in access to resources, and images of them in popular culture reveal the depth to which they are despised.

People who are old and ageing experience this sense of being 'in but not of' – redundant, unproductive, a burden. Some of them are physically removed from the rest of us, so that their not belonging, their inclusion experienced as exclusion, is very tangible and material.

Disabled people are excluded in very tangible ways, through access to public buildings, through the dominance of spoken language, through the lack of proper resources in jobs, leisure and education. Further, disability has been medicalized, seen as under the control of medical discourses which have sought to manage the individual as well as the condition. Disablement has been seen as an individual pathology, a 'personal tragedy', a defect to be remedied, a negative phenomenon which is controlled through exclusion from power of those defined as disabled (Oliver 1990). That exclusion can also include termination of pregnancy through eugenics in several countries, in an attempt to avoid contagion and racial degeneration (Madden and Humphries 1998).

The language which people use is the most revealing of the various boundaries that separate Self and Other, especially inclusive and exclusive pronouns and possessives – 'we' and 'they', 'us' and 'them', 'ours' and 'theirs'. This rhetoric of Othering dehumanizes and diminishes groups, making it easier to seize land, to exploit labour, to exert control, while minimizing complicating emotions like guilt and shame. These are legitimating techniques which have been used throughout history (Riggins 1997).

Finally, I want to point up the importance of the link between these social divisions and poverty (Leonard 1997). It is clear that within different countries, different groups of people enjoy different degrees of belonging, of inclusion, of citizenship. Some of the effects of discrimination are ameliorated by affluence and wealth, but are exacerbated by poverty.

It has been estimated that 'over 20 per cent of the world's population lives in conditions of absolute poverty, if such be defined as a situation where people cannot regularly meet their most basic subsistence needs' (Giddens 1994: 98). Significant is a dramatic increase in poverty worldwide with the growth of global capitalism, and the exploitative nature of the relationship between North and South. Within countries, the construction of particular groups as the 'Other', as 'outsiders within', has legitimated policies which deprive them of adequate income, housing and basic rights. A particularly tragic consequence is the alienation of many young people, especially young men, large numbers of them black or gay, driving increasing numbers to the ultimate act of exclusion, the taking of their own lives.

A very useful tool in this construction in some countries has been the concept of 'the underclass' (Murray 1994), especially in the USA and Britain – identified in the popular imagination as those who won't work, who exist on welfare out of choice, who are single mothers, young criminals, the feckless and the anti-social. They are all captured in that very vivid and distancing metaphor, 'the underclass'.

In some countries, notably countries of the North, attempts have been made to confront the problem of 'inclusion experienced as exclusion' through affirmative action and equal opportunities policies. Throughout the 1970s and 1980s, despite an increasingly conservative political climate, local government departments and authorities, employers, unions, universities, all appeared to recognize the unequal chances available to different sections of the population, and formulated policies for change. There is no doubt that some people were able to take advantage of this, but there were problems. Different groups were set into competition with each other for scarce resources, hierarchies of disadvantage were created, right-wing governments became increasingly hostile to the policies, and a backlash ensued from those who had been regarded as advantaged by existing social structures (see Humphries 1997a).

British social work was a very vivid example of this process, as we described in the introduction to this book, and I return to it again below. The notion of equal opportunities has not gone away, but policies have been transformed and incorporated to meet the needs of industry and the demands of social control. 'Social exclusion' is not primarily about giving opportunities to all those without, but to *target* specific groups – for example young people into employment and African-Caribbean men and Muslim women into higher education. Why? Not as a general effort towards a better deal for all, not towards a social goal of inclusion, but towards surveillance and control. As a result of this targeting, large numbers are still excluded. We should not assume that equality is an objective of such policies.

Inappropriate inclusions

I have chosen also to look at inappropriate inclusions to demonstrate the oppressive and patronizing nature of assumptions made by dominant groups, that their experience is representative of all people in a particular category everywhere. This critique is articulated within feminist theories and debates, where in challenging the universalist assumptions of knowledge constructed by men, some white feminisms have themselves adopted universalist and imperialist assumptions. Critiques from black and Third World women (e.g. Bhavnani 1991, Mohanty 1991) expose the claim to power, the hegemony in feminist theory of white Western middle-class heterosexual women, which marginalizes other Others, because their experience is assumed to be the same, but is not the same. They have been diligent about charting difference and insisting that feminist theory take account of it.

Poststructuralist insights have also informed this debate. In particular, poststructuralism identifies the categories 'woman' and 'man' as essentialist: that is, it draws attention to the ways these categories vary historically and culturally, and the importance of taking account of this diversity. Some versions of poststructuralism go too far in claiming that the categories 'woman' and 'man' are meaningless and therefore redundant (see Cealey Harrison and Hood-Williams 1998, for example).

The general point I am making is the tendency of dominant groups to assume their experience as the norm, and to theorize from it, instead of starting with an *interrogation* of their own experience in the light of the operation of power in the modern world, and their own implication in those relations of power. Experience is complex and it is diverse. Gail Lewis (1996) in her interviews with black women social workers to explore 'the black woman's experience', discovered that although the expression was used by all the women she interviewed, it was understood differently by them, in the light of their positioning in relation to other black women (e.g. those with whom they had once but no longer shared a community, clients, seniors), and also black men, white women and white men. 'The black woman's experience' was revealed as a multilayered and complex phenomenon.

A cold wind of change

These material and discursive exclusions, then, characterize the modern world. In education generally and in social work education particularly, in industrialized countries there has been a re-statement of positivist understandings of knowledge, expressed in bureaucratic and managerialist procedures, with their vocabulary of 'targets', 'packages', 'outcomes', 'competencies' (Edwards and Usher 1994, Humphries 1997b). Among teachers and social workers there is an instrumental preoccupation with outcomes and measurement, to the detriment of identification with and creative thinking alongside those excluded groups I have described. The impact of this on professional workers is a 'hegemony of resignation' (Miliband 1994), a sense of powerlessness, a loss of any belief in an alternative and a mechanistic and routinized view of the job.

The experience of social workers – diverse across different cultures – is a contradictory one – of control and surveillance on the one hand and concern for oppressed groups on the other. The contradictions are because social work cannot be disconnected from macro processes: from globalization and its impact on nation-states, from increasing poverty, from the growing chasm between rich and poor countries. It does not operate parallel and separate from these developments. Its growing role in internal immigration controls, its surveillance of the poor and the dispossessed, even the social work collaboration across countries, is on several levels linked to globalization and to the rush for profit. Market ideology and managerialism promote market values in national economic affairs and dominate all public sector activity. We must not be naive about the implication of social work and other welfare professions in all of this.

In Britain the 1980s groundswell of radicalism among communities, local authorities, social work agencies, practitioners, educators and students was reflected in education, youth work and community work, in policies and practice based on a vision of education and welfare work as agents of change, as combating racism and sexism, and as concerned primarily with challenging inequality, thus placing themselves 'in and against the state'. A unique feature of this was the involvement of the then regulating body of social work, the Central Council for the Education and Training in Social Work (CCETSW), which built a requirement for anti-racist and anti-discriminatory practice into its training regulations for qualifying social workers (CCETSW 1991). This effort was not unproblematically progressive (see Humphries 1993, 1997a). A right-wing Conservative government responded both by a ideological campaign which derided these activities as 'political correctness' (Jones 1993; Humphries 1993) and by setting about dismantling the structures which had been set up to support the anti-discriminatory policies. In social work, the training requirements were diluted in ways which fitted better with a managerialist and technicist approach (Humphries 1997b).

Although it is to be welcomed that social work was the first occupational group to make a bid explicitly claiming a role for the profession to be controversial, to make trouble with the state, it was not well grounded in a set of values which could sustain its position when trouble brewed. It was also in a contradictory role as largely a state agent. CCETSW bent itself to the wind of change, so that currently

the language of anti-discrimination is still to be found in its documentation, but the political vacuum is exposed (Humphries 1997b). Values
which challenge the roots of social systems are out of place, they sit
uneasily with what is required in modern practice, they have become
incorporated in a way that robs them of their 'dangerousness'.
Practitioners and students are not facilitated to work in ways that truly
challenge discrimination, and what they produce is often contrived,
tokenistic and meaningless.

Resources for hope

Is there, then, any hope for those other values genuinely held by the
welfare profession – social justice, an end to oppression? Is it possible
to contribute to changing the social order? How are we to proceed if
we are not to perpetuate relations of dominance? Below, I suggest
some resources for a social work praxis, for a unity of thought and
action which might be shared across professional and national boundaries. First, though, there are signals that the ideological climate
internationally is beginning to change. A crisis in capitalism is rever-
berating around the world. There are signs that the hegemony of
neo-liberalism and an uncontrolled free market is breaking down –
perhaps globalization can be tamed; perhaps inequality can be more
than just mollified; perhaps we are not after all at the mercy of nature
and the market. Martin Jacques (1998) strikes an optimistic note,
suggesting that the present global crisis offers a possibility of a sea-
change in attitudes, that the laissez-faire mentality that has dominated
for the past twenty-five years is now under serious threat all around
the globe, that it is possible to control what we have been told is
uncontrollable.

The social work and welfare professions should take comfort from
this, recognize that what they are required to do is not inevitable, and
seek for ways to contribute to this 'sea-change'.

Valuing subjugated knowledges

First, we must root the intellectual base of social work in more than
technical and managerial values, in more than common-sense understandings and slogans about injustice. Part of that is the recognition of
knowledges which have been excluded from scientific discourses and
largely from professional discourses – low status knowledge, subjugated knowledge, 'Other' knowledge.

This starts with an understanding of how people come to be known through discourses of racialization, gender, sexuality, disablement. The categories attached to these processes are not simply descriptive, they are *contested social constructions*. At the heart of struggles over meaning within these discourses is the issue of identity and the ability to name the self. Social work is engaged in the bureaucratic naming, in classifying, in labelling, in categorizing people all the time. Many of these categories are informed by and contribute to racialized sexualized gendered epistemologies of the Other, not in any universal and trans-historical truth. Yet they are employed daily in decision-making, often in unreflected-upon and uncritical ways.

Often excluded from the academy are those knowledges which represent a self-naming of subjugated groups and peoples. Dyer says, 'the claim to power is the claim to speak for the commonality of humanity' (1997: 2). We need to recognize that the universals of a discourse of 'justice' and 'emancipation' are themselves socially constructed. They are culturally relative and are not necessarily shared, even as ideals (Leonard 1997). Other notions of human welfare, silenced by Western colonialism, speak to show that it is possible to think differently than many of us have previously thought, perceive the world differently, and therefore act differently. Can we enter a process where we can arrive at some agreed values rather than assumed values, which Leonard calls 'universal by consent' (1997: 28)?

Culturally produced conceptions of welfare include not only Western models but African, Aboriginal, Asian. There are black epistemologies, feminisms, sexualities and theories of disablement which need to be examined and interrogated in the attempt to pull ourselves out of the hegemony of resignation and construct a knowledge base which offers an alternative to the narrow surveillance and managerialist culture affecting social work in many societies.

An interactive universalism

My second resource comes out of the critique I mentioned earlier, which comes from black and Third World women and from poststructuralisms. Poststructuralisms advocate a jettisoning of grand narratives as a theoretical base for understanding the world – universal theories based on class, gender, 'race', for example – and advocate an emphasis on difference, the particular, the local. They argue that there are too many historical, geographical and cultural variables for these general theories to make sense any more. It is an approach which risks a relativism which could undermine a shared sense of struggle against exploitation and inequality across the world. Emphasis on difference can be used by national governments as a relatively safe, money-saving rationale for small-scale adjustments which could fragment populations into ever smaller 'communities of interest', thus weakening collective resistance (Leonard 1997).

The insights of poststructuralism are important warnings against homogenizing influences and the dangers of theorizing inequality at a general level, but they go too far in condemning such a project as unproductive. There is enough evidence of cross-cultural continuity of poverty, of women's subordinate position, of racism, to warrant some general conclusions. But a richer understanding of diversity, of difference, can inform strategic questions of a role for contemporary social work. The adoption of what has been called variously a concept of 'common difference' (Doyal 1995: 4), or a 'differential universalism' (Lister 1997: 90) or an 'interactive universalism' (Benhabib 1992: 3), catches both the commonalities across cultures and the plurality of human interests. If social work across countries is concerned with social justice, the alliances and coalitions we form would do well to focus on these ideas of commonality and difference, and work on translating them into action in social work contexts.

Internationalism

Finally, I think what has been implied in what I have been saying is a concept of internationalism as a resource for a social work praxis. A number of writers on citizenship and in the social policy field are emphasizing the importance of an international perspective (Lister 1997). The United Nations has warned that the growing gulf between rich and poor countries can only be tackled by a 'new international solidarity' (United Nations 1996). Is there a role for social work in helping to prevent the perpetuation of domination and exclusion? In many ways the structures are in place through the various collaborations which have been set up. These include collaborations introduced by the European Union through *Erasmus*, *Tempus*, *Leonardo*. They include potential links through DYFYD. Networks already exist with a concern about, for example, racism and anti-semitism and disability internationally. How many of those collaborations have as a central concern the impact of globalization and its state of crisis; the implications of immigration controls, both external and internal; the myriad internal exclusions which operate at both discursive and material levels; the inappropriate assimilations and incorporation of marginalized groups which serve to reinforce their Otherness? How many are seeking to engage with the silenced and dismissed knowledges of subjugated peoples?

Of course, social workers cannot single-handedly change international law, or the global market or the legal status of individuals. But they have a responsibility to look beyond the confines of everyday practices, beyond the individualism and the managerialism, make sense of what is happening in the wider world, and make their contribution to the changes. They can do this through national and international communities of social work organizations at both educational and practice levels, with negotiated ideals of social justice far more explicitly part of their agenda than they are now. The ability to effect change in the modern world must go beyond group differences and national boundaries, and depends on the building of international coalitions, alliances and networks across professional boundaries and with those people directly affected by exclusive practices: alliances which do not seek to impose a dominant model of justice or well-being, but approach their work together modestly, and which foster an attitude of dialogue and a willingness to be influenced by each other. Such a project would reassert social work's right and role to be controversial and challenging instead of malleable and compliant, and would be a sign of hope for a better world. The global economic convulsions signal that the opportunities are here to be grasped.

Note

1   Incidentally, we have here a good example of action which resists unjust practices. A partnership of probation officers, partners of prisoners and local immigration advice services raised the profile of double punishment to bring it to visibility, and campaigned to end the practice.

References

Benhabib, S. (1992) *Situating the Self*, Cambridge: Polity Press.
Bhavnani, K.K. (1991) 'What's power got to do with it? Empowerment and social research', in I. Parker and J. Shotter (eds), *Deconstructing Social Psychology*, London: Routledge.
Castles, S. and Miller, M.J. (1993) *The Age of Migration: International Population Movements in the Modern World*, Basingstoke: Macmillan.
CCETSW (1991) *Rules and Requirements for the Diploma in Social Work*, Paper 30, London: CCETSW.
Cealey Harrison, W. and Hood-Williams, J. (1998) 'More varieties than Heinz: social categories and sociality in Humphries, Hammersley and beyond', *Sociological Research Online*, 3(1), http://www.socresonline.org.uk/socresonline/3/1/8.html

Cohen, S. and Hayes, D. (1998) *They Make You Sick: Essays on Immigration Controls and Health*, Manchester: Greater Manchester Immigration Aid Unit and Manchester Metropolitan University.

Cohen, S., Hayes, D., Humphries, B. and Sime, C. (1997) *Immigration Controls and Health*, Manchester: Greater Manchester Immigration Aid Unit and Manchester Metropolitan University.

Commission of the European Communities (1992) *Combating Social Exclusion, Fostering Integration*, Brussels: Commission of the European Communities (DGV).

——(1993) 'Towards a Europe of solidarity: combating social exclusion', *Social Europe*, 4.

Doyal, L. (1995) *What Makes Women Sick?: Gender and the Political Economy of Health*, London: Macmillan.

Dyer, R. (1997) *White*, London: Routledge.

Edwards, R. and Usher, R. (1994) 'Disciplining the subject: the power of competence', *Studies in the Education of Adults*, 26(1), 1–14.

Giddens, A. (1994) *Beyond Left and Right*, Stanford, CA: Stanford University Press.

GMIAU (1998) *Campaign Against Double Punishment* (second edition), Manchester: Greater Manchester Immigration Aid Unit.

Humphries, B. (1993) 'Are you or have you ever been ...?' *Social Work Education*, 12(3), 6–8.

——(1997a) 'The dismantling of anti-discrimination in British social work: a view from social work education', *International Social Work*, 40(3), 289–301.

——(1997b) 'Reading social work: competing discourses in the Rules and Requirements for the Diploma in Social Work', *British Journal of Social Work*, 27(5), 641–8.

——(1998) 'The baby and the bath water: Hammersley, Cealey Harrison and Hood-Williams and the emancipatory research debate', *Sociological Research Online*, 3(1), http://www.socresonline.org.uk/socresonline/3/1/9.html

Jacques, M. (1998) 'J'accuse: Tony Blair goes on trial', *Marxism Today*, special edition, 20 October 1998.

Jones, C. (1993) 'Distortion and demonization: the Right and anti-racist social work education', *Social Work Education*, 12(3), 9–16.

Leonard, P. (1997) *Postmodern Welfare: Reconstructing an Emancipatory Project*, London: Sage.

Lewis, G. (1996) 'Situated voices: black women's experience and social work', *Feminist Review*, 53 (Summer), 24–56.

Lister, R. (1997) *Citizenship: Feminist Perspectives*, London: Macmillan.

Madden, M. and Humphries, B. (1998), *The Construction of Social Research Knowledge*, Manchester: Manchester Metropolitan University Department of Applied Community Studies/Sage.

Miliband, R. (1994) *Thirty years of the Socialist Register*, London: Merlin Press, 1–19.

Mohanty, C.T. (1991) 'Under Western eyes: feminist scholarship and colonial discourses', in C.T. Mohanty, A. Russo and L. Torres (eds), *Third World Women and the Politics of Feminism*, Bloomington, IA: Indiana University Press.

Murray, C. (1994) *Underclass: The Crisis Deepens*, London: IEA Health and Welfare Unit, Choice in Welfare Series no. 20.

Oliver, M. (1990) *The Politics of Disablement*, London: Macmillan.

Riggins, S.H. (ed.) (1997) *The Language and Politics of Exclusion: Others in Discourse*, Thousand Oaks, CA, and London: Sage.

Riley, D. (1988) *Am I That Name?* London: Macmillan.

Sivanandan, A. (1993) 'Beyond statewatching', in T. Bunyan (ed.), *Statewatching the New Europe*, London: Statewatch.

United Nations (1991) 'The World's Women (1970–1990): Trends and Statistics', *Social Statistics and Indicators*, Series K, no. 8, New York: UN.

——(1996) *The Human Development Report*, 1996 and 1994, UNDP.

Yuval Davis, N. (1991) 'The citizenship debate: women, ethnic processes and the state', *Feminist Review*, 39, 58–68.

7 Critical professionals and reflective practice

The experience of women practitioners in health, welfare and education

Mary Issitt

Over the last two decades reflective practice has become integrated as a goal and process in professional education and development, influenced primarily by the work of Donald Schon. According to Michael Eraut, *The Reflective Practitioner* (Schon 1983) 'has probably been the most quoted book on professional expertise during the last ten years' (Eraut 1994: 149). One of the attractions of the concept is its flexibility and applicability in a wide range of professional contexts. However, this results in it meaning different things to different people, and its adoption is claimed by those with different ideologies and often competing intentions as to its use.

In this chapter I explore some of the different ways of seeing reflective practice, using a feminist perspective to highlight problems with the concept together with possibilities for progressive practice. An important concern will be to identify ways of thinking about and approaching reflective practice that can lead to the development of 'critical intelligence' which Janet Batsleer and Beth Humphries believe enables practitioners to address the dilemmas of trying to work against injustice, within market-oriented organizational structures that often perpetuate inequalities and division between people (see the Introduction to this book).

I draw upon different accounts and perspectives on reflective practice gleaned from research I undertook through interviews and focus groups with 34 women during 1997 and 1998.[1] The research participants were accessed through existing feminist, community and education networks covering a wide spectrum of occupations with representation from both managerial and grass-roots levels of practice. The age range was from late twenties to mid-fifties, with the majority being in the 31–40 age group. While eight participants were from minority ethnic backgrounds, the majority defined their ethnicity as white and European. Three of these were white Jewish women. Two participants described themselves as disabled, and in the course of the research five women referred to their sexual orientation as lesbian. Between them, these women had extensive experience as professionals working in education, health, housing, social services and youth and community work, often having moved between these different sectors. As well as their various paid work they had or were now undertaking, between them they had been, or were currently involved in, over 150 different kinds of voluntary activities.

During the chapter I report their perspectives and experience of reflective practice and identify key issues that I hope will enable the practitioner to distinguish a critical approach from other models with which they may be presented. As a feminist who has worked or been a volunteer/activist in the human service contexts represented by the women participants, I feel that feminism provides one way, which is accessible to me, whereby I can begin to gain a critical understanding, and this is considered in more detail in the next part of the chapter.

A feminist approach to researching reflective practice

Feminism is a contested discipline, and Williams (1996) shows how the feminism of the 1970s which stressed the commonality between women has been challenged:

> Feminism based on black, lesbian and disabled politics has pointed to the need to deconstruct the category 'woman' in order to understand the complex and inter-connected range of identities and subject positions through which women's experiences are constituted, as well as the way these also change over time and place.
>
> (Williams 1996: 69)

Some research participants (mainly black women and one white, lesbian woman) felt that 'womanism' was a term that they could more closely identify with, echoing Martin and Webster's (1994) view that: 'Womanism is a term that some of us feel we can take ownership of because it is non-eurocentric and non-western in its application and it is therefore more acceptable to us' (Martin and Webster 1994: 4).

One black woman participant felt that feminism and womanism were two sides of the same coin; as Alice Walker has commented, 'feminism is to womanism as purple is to lavender' (1992: xii).

In undertaking the research with women who regarded themselves as influenced by feminism/womanism, I was not seeking to identify an overarching model of feminist reflective practice that obscured different identities and experience. While I was concerned to explore shared notions of the relationship of anti-oppressive practice to reflective practice, I was also interested to find out from participants about what Williams (1996: 70) calls 'different political understandings of the notions of difference' and how these impacted on the concept. I felt that a feminist lens would enable me to engage critically with reflective practice for the following reasons:

1   Although the analysis may vary, a common thread running through feminism and womanism (apart from liberal feminism, Williams 1989) is an understanding of power relations and recognition of oppression in respect of gender, race, class, sexuality and disability;
2   This translates into a value-base which, in the feminism that interests me, is concerned to make a difference in people's lives (Stanley and Wise 1993). It is not merely concerned with academic debate, although the importance of debate is recognized;
3   Feminist analysis has made a significant contribution to critical perspectives on social policy (Pascall 1997; George and Wilding 1994) and to practice in human service work (Butler and Wintram 1991; Ernst and Goodison 1981; Langan and Day 1992).
4   There are potentially a number of features that reflective practice shares with feminism and I wanted to explore these further. I was concerned that the discourses of reflective practice and feminism had run parallel to each other, yet each had made significant contributions to the critique of positivist epistemology and methodology, and contained recognition of the significance of reflexivity for those in human service work (Issitt 1999).

Reflective practice: its popularity and problems

Before considering the research findings, I will outline some of the key features of reflective practice, based upon the work of Donald Schon (1930–97). He argued for many years that there had been a crisis in professional knowledge which left professionals ill equipped to meet the demands of practice. While there have been a variety of tensions and conflicts of different origin, a major problem that professionals have faced is the dominance of positivist epistemology in their education. This inevitably leads to an overemphasis on a technically rational model of professionalism, which proposes 'blueprints' for problem-solving that are often not feasible in the practice context. Professionals frequently operate within 'indeterminate zones of practice' – unique situations that require a mixture of complex judgements, decision-making and action. A 'technically rational' approach might be inviting, but it often means excluding aspects of the problem and bringing about a partial solution.

To be really effective, the practitioner has to be spontaneous and creative in her problem-solving by using 'intelligence in action' (tacit knowledge) which includes 'recognition and judgement as well as the exercise of ordinary physical skills' (Schon 1992: 56). She engages in 'reflection-in-action', a form of 'on-the-spot inquiry' (ibid.: 57) to integrate tacit and explicit knowledge, experience and 'professional artistry' in 'an action-present – a stretch of time within which it is still possible to make a difference to the outcomes of the action' (ibid.: 58). Reflective practice not only involves 'reflection-in-action' in the 'action-present', but 'reflection-on-action' after the event as part of an understanding of, and preparation for, further action and professional development.

One of the reasons that reflective practice may have become so popular is that it offers a means of countering the 'downgrading of critical analysis' (Gould 1996: 4) which has followed the re-framing of human service professions in terms of occupational standards of competence. Many argue that this paradigm shift towards the workplace as the preferred location in which learning is demonstrated, assessed and developed leads to an overemphasis on performance (Hyland 1995). For Jones and Moore (1995): 'The competency model has been constructed not because it is good to think with but because it is good to use within the very particular policy context in which it has been active over recent years' (Jones and Moore 1995: 84).

This policy context, ushered in by the Thatcherite reforms of the 1980s, claiming to end bureaucracy and promote more efficient and effective services in the public sector, required a profound culture change led by a new managerialism (Clarke and Newman 1997). A renegotiation of working relationships at all levels of human service work has ensued as the new roles of purchaser and provider have been created and become embedded, and the thrusting language of the market-place adopted. The new managerialist agenda emphasized competence-based assessment in the workplace, to assure that providers will have the individuals, within a 'competent' organization to deliver the required contract outcomes (Hodkinson and Issitt 1995; Issitt 1996).

The restructuring of welfare and education means that human

service professionals have had to re-evaluate every aspect of their work: what they do, how they do it and how they think about it. This has often led to anxiety as 'old' ways of working were seen to be undervalued (Dalley *et al.* 1991) in favour of a prevailingly task-centred reductionist model of competence (Issitt 1996, 1999; Gould 1996) which is often justified with 'a veneer of objectivity' (Issitt and Woodward 1992). However, the definition and execution of competence in human service occupations reflects an anti-collectivist ideology concerned to redefine the nature of the professional role (Humphries 1997; Issitt 1995). In social work this has been part of a process to undermine professionals' fundamental concerns to tackle inequalities in society by labelling it as 'political correctness' (Dominelli 1996). Reflective practice has been invoked as an alternative method-ology that could enable practitioners 'to challenge the normative context of practice, and to be non-defensive and adaptive learners within a constantly evolving professional environment' (Gould 1996: 4).

In professions such as nursing, social work and teaching there has been a concern to promote reflective practice (Palmer *et al.* 1994; Yelloly and Henkel 1995; Zeichner 1994) as both a goal and a process in the development of autonomous professionals who can synthesize theory and practice in order to maximize their capacity for creativity in their work. Thus the reflective practitioner

> who recognizes the limits of professional knowledge and action, builds in a cycle of critical reflection to maximize the capacity for critical thought and produces a sense of professional freedom and a connection with rather than a distance from clients.
>
> (Pietroni 1995: 43)

Schon's approach to reflective practice appears to fit within hermeneutics, placing 'subjectivity at centre stage' (Thompson 1995: 44). Its recognition of the subjective engagement of the professional in her practice celebrating creativity and 'professional artistry' human service professions may be more appealing than competence models that emphasize mere functional performance. Schon's work has been criticized for 'making little or no reference' to 'the socio-political factors which can have a major impact on the context in which learning and practice take place' (Thompson 1995: 78). But Ecclestone suggests that critical enquiry can be part of reflective practice, enabling the practitioner to 'examine the contradictions between their own values and beliefs and the dominant social and institutional norms which govern their practice' (Ecclestone 1996: 155).

The flexibility of reflective practice leaves it open to appropriation by 'different stakeholders to serve different educational and social purposes' (Ecclestone 1996: 154). This occurs 'when issues of values and ideology are severed from the debate about different principles' (ibid.). Thus, in spite of Schon's trenchant critique of technical rationality, 'a superficial reconciliation of principles and practice' (ibid.) means that, paradoxically, reflective practice may be claimed by programmes that promote a narrow technicist approach and 'is most clearly manifested in NVQs[2] where any reflection would focus on how well practitioners are achieving predefined outcomes' (ibid.: 15).

The teacher education courses Ecclestone cites encompass those concerned to respond effectively and efficiently to the market, those involving social accountability and risk-taking, and those whose orientation is towards personal learning and development through reflection. All claim to be training their students to be reflective practitioners, and, following Ball (1994), she argues that the term becomes a mantra that is recited as a substitute for real enquiry in contrast with an educational tradition through which reflection:

> effectively challenges the thinking about events, circumstances and philosophies which constitute and value the status quo ... [it] is seen as a means of emancipation and empowerment, a vehicle for allowing both teacher educators and teachers to take control of the environment and circumstances in which they and students learn.
>
> (Knowles 1986: 82)

In order to use reflection in the way that Knowles proposes, there is a need for a critical stance that interrogates concepts such as 'emancipation' and 'empowerment' (Baistow 1994/5; Clarke and Newman 1997), recognizing their contested nature. It would also mean understanding and acting upon the factors that prevent professionals and clients, teachers and students from taking control of their environment and circumstances.

Bearing in mind the potentially different interpretations of reflective practice, in the next part of the chapter I draw upon views expressed by women who participated in my research to explore the problems and possibilities for operating as a feminist reflective practitioner within the current service context. An important issue to consider is how the criticality, which comes from feminism and womanism, enables reflection to go beyond the confines of the individual's work, to interrogate the dynamic existing between the subjective experience of practice and the professional and political contexts in which the practice takes place. To facilitate dialogue with the research participants I used statements that drew upon Schon's work described above, together with the quotation from Pietroni (1995) noted earlier, and statements about feminism and values underpinning anti-oppressive practice.

Participants' understanding of reflective practice

Reflective practice involves individual reflection and personal evaluation

It was interesting that, although the concept of 'reflective practice' was something that participants immediately identified with and for which a number were able to offer their own definitions, very few had read the literature on reflective practice, or had not done so for several years. However, a common view was expressed that implied that reflective practice was very clearly linked with experiential learning and development (Tsang 1998).

Participants described a systematic educative process, involving constant evaluation of current practice and modifying future practice, 'understanding my own actions, recognizing diversity, moving forward and challenge ... if ever I didn't feel nervous about going into a teaching session then I'm not doing it properly'.

As one woman showed, it links clearly with notions of being 'research-minded':

> I think about things in terms of reflecting on what I have done. I try and use that cycle ... you do it, you write about it, you consider it and let that inform how you work and how you plan. In part like an evaluation cycle.

Reflective practice was something that could happen at different stages within one's personal life, even in childhood, or at different occupational levels.

A number of women working in training and education were involved in recognizing and developing reflective practice in others. One who is now a university lecturer, formerly an NVQ assessor in social care, observed that some people were 'natural reflective practitioners' and this transformed the way that they approached 'even mundane tasks' and had deeper significance for those for whom they were caring. Another uses reflective learning in her current role as an

NVQ assessor to encourage candidates in 'identifying their strengths ... their weaknesses, and areas they need to work on ... it's like an ongoing practice ... even when they get their certificate at the end, I'm always saying to them you never stop learning'.

An adult education tutor incorporates reflection into all her learning programmes and sees this as integral to her own feminist reflective practice encouraging the women tutors whose work she co-ordinates to meet regularly to share their experiences and feelings about what they are doing: 'So for them it is constantly about having assumptions challenged, lots about dealing with women ... and often black or working-class women.'

An important issue was to enable practitioners to become aware of their own reflection so that it becomes visible and systematic. A community worker described how this happens on a project to enable experienced practitioners to become professionally qualified as youth and community workers through a work-based accreditation process.

> Reflective practice is actually something that everybody does but it's something we are not necessarily aware of, that's what you were saying about Schon ... reflection in action ... reflection on action ... and that happens. Just to pull that out and ... see for them-selves what they are doing in situations and how they are actually adjusting the objectives ... how they are then transferring that then to other situations ... that's one of the benefits of the process.

The non-elitist approach to reflective practice shown in the quotes above contrasts with the argument, which sometimes appears in the professional literature, that reflective practice can only be aspired to by those who are not 'novices' in their professional work, and that this can only come some years after the completion of training programmes (Eraut 1994). A Principal Youth Officer was emphatic that it should not be seen as 'something rarefied, something special'.

Another woman summed reflective practice up very aptly as follows, acknowledging the complexity of interactions at all levels of human service work: 'It is something that is a formulation of both knowledge and experience ... quite an advanced concept ... however, it doesn't necessarily live only in an advanced place.'

Reflection not only operates at the individual level but also is a group process

One woman made the link between the individual and group dimensions of reflective practice as follows:

> Some reflective practice you do on your own, you don't need to take it anywhere. But other bits you think … I do need to discuss that with other people … I want to be able to get the benefit of their views on that … we do reflective practice at lots of different levels and lots of different scenarios.

Reflective practice involves group discussion and networking through feminist/womanist and other networks and may feature as an important part of different cultures. One African-Caribbean woman likened reflective practice to the act of 'reasoning' that takes place among groups of Jamaican people when you:

> Check out the position you are coming from, think about the position other people are coming from, does it hold water … if not, why not, and that starts within your family and through your friends … it's a whole that informs and influences the position that you take.

Sometimes reflective practice came through action. For some this was political action outside the work context, but it could involve working collectively as part of a cohesive team in which discussion and support was an accepted part of the work. One woman describes a situation in the mid-1980s, when she worked with a women's health team: 'So our day-to-day bread and butter is this theoretical intellectual practical debate, every single working day, and that validates in a way.'

The sense of group involvement, enthusiasm, commitment and dynamism which is expressed in the above quotation is echoed by others. A former probation officer described how in the mid-1980s she had been able to do creative work with women around community development and domestic violence. This involvement built upon her understanding of feminism, developed as a mature student on a postgraduate social work course. However, as the populist and New Right agenda for law and order prioritized retribution and punishment over rehabilitation (Jordan and Arnold 1995) the emphasis in the probation officer's role shifted from that of welfare to control. This former probation officer still maintained her links with women's groups in the sphere of domestic violence and criminal justice, and as a result knew what was happening in people's lives, remaining in touch in the way that Pietroni's (1995) quote suggests. However, she feels that the space for this kind of developmental preventive work was no longer a legitimate part of the probation officer's role following the Criminal Justice Act 1991. Thus: 'It was really hard to do any reflective practice because I think it got to the point, it was literally just a conveyor belt. You write PSRs [pre-sentence reports], you're not here to be reflective practitioners.'

Reflective practice needs the right conditions in order to flourish

As the above example shows, operating creatively as a reflective practitioner may not fit with the current policy context. Reflective practice as a model for learning and development implies that the professional has an openness to improving her practice. However, the regulation and finance-driven accountability required by the new managerialism has implications for being open about identifying better ways of working which would involve sharing personal vulnerability. While for one woman, 'my impulse is always to let someone know what lessons I have learnt, even in a competitive situation', many felt that reflective practice was not valued in the current policy and practice context.

One woman demonstrated how her personal and professional value-base was in conflict with the political climate of her work setting. The honest evaluation and reflection that she incorporates within her role is discouraged by management attitudes which are driven by the outcomes focus of the quasi-market situation in which she works. She has to edit from her work-reports questions about why she may not have achieved targets in a particular aspect of her work. She feels that the quality systems operate against her in this way: 'It's not about doing things properly – it's about gathering the paperwork'.

Many felt that in their current or immediately previous paid work context, there was not room for reflective practice, which might be time-consuming and slow down 'production'. Reflection that at the personal and professional level is a necessity becomes a luxury, and 'you can't get together with your colleagues'. This was illustrated by the members of a focus group of community workers who participated in the research. Although they worked in the same city and had met in the past as a women's network, this was not now sanctioned within their work contexts. They welcomed the opportunity to get together to reflect on issues that they saw as relevant to their practice, which the 'external' justification of participation in the research gave.

Thus the time that is required for reflection is not available in the current market-orientated world of human service work. For some it becomes 'invisible' and takes place as a private moment of 'reflection-in' or 'on-action', or through more structured diary-writing in their own time. When reflection is not integrated into the work situation then the service loses out, as the emotional aspects of human service work need to be dealt with at the personal and professional level. Two participants contrasted the non-managerial supervision in a health promotion setting which had been superseded by a different outcomes-oriented managerialist model. This had discouraged reflective practice, being 'much more task-orientated rather than providing emotional support to you, and I think we've lost out because I found that really good for reflecting'.

A clear message that comes across from the participants is that reflective practice which provides emotional support should not be about unproductive self-indulgent navel-gazing that does not lead anywhere other than 'analysis-paralysis'.

Reflective practice is challenging

All agreed that reflective practice was not an easy option to pursue for a variety of reasons. At the organizational level it may be challenging to what one woman called the 'here and now answer' that the prevailing contract culture often required. Because the reflective practitioner might ask questions requiring longer-term solutions than the new managerialist culture, discussed by Clarke and Newman (1997), allows, it is often dismissed as unproductive and time-consuming.

Some research participants talked about the need for reflective practice for both the individual and the group to take place in 'safe spaces', with people being able to share and get to know each other. A number were emphatic that this wasn't a cosy space in which to hide from reality. It was 'safe' in that it provided an arena in which to be challenged into new ways of thinking and to build solidarity that could translate into both understanding and action. This relates to the concern of a number of the research participants that reflective practice involved an understanding of power relationships, and linking the personal, professional and societal levels was central. Rogers (1978) provides a summary of politics as:

the process of gaining, using, sharing, or relinquishing power control or decision-making. It is the process of the highly complex interactions and effects of these elements as they exist in relationship between persons, between a person and a group, or between groups.

(Rogers 1978: 5)

Therefore, reflective practitioners had to acknowledge their own personal power, and also that of others who may have a management role in relation to them. One woman recalled a situation in which she now realizes she was constantly undermined by her manager; reflection became a very negative thing for her, so consequently it became centred on, ' "What crap I am" rather than, "Did I do that well?" ... and what is the learning from that?' The responses of women participants endorsed McNay's (1992: 56) view that:

Using power relations as a unifying concept necessitates an exploration of the dimensions of power whenever we consider explanations of social issues. It may not be necessary or appropriate to reject particular theories, but rather to understand how being set in a wider context of power would change their meaning.

This analysis enables reflective practitioners to examine their own personal power, the limits within which it can realistically operate, and the interface between the personal, professional and wider societal dimensions of power. It can provide some protection from internalizing blame at the personal level for problems that required a wider solution. For many, identifying as a feminist or a womanist was central to this process. As one woman said, 'I don't think you can, as a feminist, not look at the wider context because there would be a contradiction where you located the problem'. She considered it 'bizarre' that anyone could claim to be a reflective practitioner without taking account of the political context.

Reflection and anti-oppressive practice

The women who participated in this research show that reflective practice as a concept and process has meaning and utility for them, and the comments reported above show the dynamic between feminism or womanism and reflective practice. For some, reflection provided the way into being a critical professional who could understand and act upon the personal, professional and political dimensions of practice.

For others, it seemed that feminist or womanist reflexivity provided the critical base for practice that is reflective. Feminism and reflective practice is so closely interwoven for some participants that when the capacity for reflection is denied the practice becomes impoverished.

Although the research inquiry was concerned with the influence of feminist and womanist perspectives, the view was clearly expressed by women participants that this perspective should be part of anti-oppressive practice. Critical reflection committed to anti-oppressive practice provides a way into tackling dimensions of power that operates at the ideological level to maintain the control of dominant groups in society (Spicker 1995). For some it was anti-oppressive practice, which is concerned to challenge unequal power relationships (Hopton 1997; Issitt 1995), that provided the key mechanism for analysing power relations in human service work.

This involved a critique of feminism, acknowledging the divisions and differences within it referred to earlier (Williams 1996), and recognizing that while feminism may claim to promote co-operation and sharing it could also act to exclude. Thus, the view was expressed in the research that a label such as feminism needs to be understood, as it may not impact upon the lives of working-class women and those from different cultures, for whom other identities may be more significant. One woman said that if you used the term 'feminism' to her mother,

> she'll wonder what you're talking about but she's a good role model in fighting barriers and oppression ... from a personal point of view I just challenge things. I'm always challenging barriers and attitudes and stereotypes ... but I don't think about it just as a woman ... I'm having to do it just to survive ... not just within my own community but within the world of work ... I suppose I think of myself as being black before I think of myself as being a woman ... because that's the obvious barrier.

This point is also raised by another woman who wanted positive change for women but felt that:

> the issue for me is that the other baggage, if you like, that I come with ... from a black perspective having that debate, which is more important, being black or being a woman ... that debate is ongoing ... that is where I have a problem with feminism ... that it doesn't take account of those considerations ... it becomes a gender-specific issue ... and for me that's not enough ... I cannot divorce myself from black men.

What does feminist anti-oppressive reflective practice mean?

The synthesis of anti-oppressive and reflective practice is particularly demanding; one woman felt that 'it actually requires you to do two jobs at once. It requires you to be a reflective practitioner and be anti-oppressive about what you have done'. The experience of the women who participated in the research shows that it has particular benefits both for the services they are working in and how they feel about their work.

The research shows that instead of being presented as a new approach to human service work, reflective practice can build profitably upon existing theories and methodology within human services. It requires an openness and predisposition to lifelong learning, linking with professionals adopting 'dialogical' approaches with service users, being concerned to accredit and build upon the experience and capability of communities. It involves the practitioner taking responsibility to promote person-centred experiential learning for themselves and with others, the development of research-mindedness and the practitioner as action researcher (Hart and Bond 1995).

Moreover, reflective practice is not just about improving technical ability, but also involves dealing with and bringing about change. An anti-oppressive feminist/womanist approach would seek to connect the personal, professional and the political dimensions with reflection as a systematic activity. The following key points are an attempt to synthesize the feedback from the research with wider analysis and are presented as a basis for further discussion and development.

The reflective practitioner – an anti-oppressive approach
- recognizes that professional knowledge is imperfect and can always be improved;
- realizes that technical expertise is necessary but that there are not formulaic answers to complex questions – Schon's 'indeterminate zones of practice';
- operates within an integrated personal/professional/political value-base which uses an analysis of power relations and commitment to anti-oppressive practice, that seeks to understand and change the social and political context affecting practice;
- 'builds in a cycle of critical reflection to maximize the capacity for critical thought, and produces a sense of professional freedom and a connection with rather than a distance from clients' (Pietroni 1995: 43);

- needs a safe, supportive environment in which to honestly reflect and practice;
- listens and learns from ways of reflecting in different cultures and groups.

Reflection does not only involve looking back, i.e. 'reflection-on-action', but also 'reflection in action', using knowledge, skills and past experience to respond creatively to new situations in the here and now. Reflection is a collaborative as well as an individual process, based upon dialogue and support.

Markets, inequality, social exclusion and reflective practice

The experience of women who have participated in this research has generally shown that many would express a commitment to the feminist/womanist reflective practice approach suggested above, as this enables them to critically evaluate and get satisfaction from what they do. However, they have generally experienced the markets in education, health and welfare as hostile environments in which the outcomes focus does not allow the time for attention to reflective processes that challenge the dominant, positivist/behaviourist underpinnings of the new managerialism of the market. Those with the most positive experience have managed to create spaces through their support networks or by moving into new occupational areas that are more receptive to the challenge of anti-oppressive, reflective practice. Clearly, this is not an option for most people, and for many reflection has become a private affair that is about survival.

As the government embarks on what it claims is the most far-reaching reform of the welfare state since the 1940s, multi-agency approaches to tackling the causes of inequality in education, health and employment are now being promoted. Partnerships between government, local agencies and individuals are the order of the day (Department of Health 1998). The fact that equality is now on the agenda, yet the market orientation of the state remains much the same, means that feminist/womanist reflective practitioners will need all the criticality and energy they can muster in order to determine whether the language of equality and opportunity is merely being adopted to sweeten unpalatable policies. It remains to be seen how far a model of reflective practice that seeks to challenge power relations can be sustained.

Acknowledgements

I very much appreciate both the contribution of the 34 women who have participated in the interviews and focus groups and the work of Doreen Speakman, who did the initial categorization of the data.

I would like to thank Janet Batsleer and Beth Humphries and participants in the social divisions and research network at Manchester Metropolitan University, also Ian Stronach, all of whose comments on an earlier draft helped me to reframe this chapter.

Notes

1   This research forms part of a project to inquire into 'Feminism, Competence and Reflective Practice', supported through the Nuffield Foundation's Small Grants Scheme.
2   NVQs refer in England and Wales to National Vocational Qualifications, which in Scotland are called Scottish Vocational Qualifications.

References

Baistow, K. (1994/5) 'Liberation and regulation? Some paradoxes of empowerment', *Critical Social Policy* 42 (Winter), 34–46.
Ball, S.J. (1994) 'Intellectuals or technicians: the urgent role of theory in educational studies', annual address to the Standing Conference for Studies in Education, RSA, London, 4 November. Cited in K. Ecclestone (1996) 'The reflective practitioner: mantra or model for emancipation?', *Studies in the Education of Adults* 28(2), 146–61.
Butler, S. and Wintram, C. (1991) *Feminist Groupwork*, London: Sage.
Clarke, J. and Newman, J. (1997) *The Managerial State*, London: Sage.
Dalley, G. with Baldwin, S., Carr-Hill, R., Hennessey, S. and Smedley, E. (1991) *Quality Management Initiatives in the NHS, Strategic Approaches to Improving Quality*, QMI Series no. 3, York: University of York Centre for Health Economics.
Department of Health (1998) *Our Healthier Nation*, Cm3852, London: HMSO.
Dominelli, L. (1996) 'Deprofessionalizing social work: anti-oppressive practice, competencies and postmodernism', in *British Journal of Social Work*, 26, 153–75.
Ecclestone, K. (1996) 'The reflective practitioner: mantra or model for emancipation?' *Studies in the Education of Adults* 28(2), 146–61.
Eraut, M. (1994) *Developing professional knowledge and competence*, London: Falmer Press.
Ernst, S. and Goodison, S. (1981) *In Our Own Hands: A Book of Self-Help Therapy*, London: The Women's Press.

132   *Mary Issitt*

George, V. and Wilding, P. (1994) *Welfare and Ideology*, Hemel Hempstead: Harvester Wheatsheaf.

Gould, N. (1996) 'Introduction: social work education and the crisis in the professions', in N. Gould and I. Taylor (eds) *Reflective Learning for Social Work*, Aldershot: Arena.

Hart, L. and Bond, M. (1995) *Action Research for Health and Social Care*, Buckingham: Open University.

Hodkinson, P. and Issitt, M. (1995) *The Challenge of Competence: Vocationalism through Education and Training*, London: Cassell.

Hopton, J. (1997) 'Anti-discriminatory practice and anti-oppressive practice: a radical humanist psychology perspective', *Critical Social Policy*, 17(3), 52, 47–62.

Humphries, B. (1997) 'Reading social work: competing discourses in the Rules and Requirements for the Diploma in Social Work', *British Journal of Social Work*, 27, 641–58.

Hyland, T. (1995) 'Behaviourism and the meaning of competence', in P. Hodkinson and M. Issitt (eds), *The Challenge of Competence: Professionalism Through Vocational Education and Training*, London: Cassell, 44–57.

Issitt, M. (1995) 'Competence, professionalism and equal opportunities', in P. Hodkinson and M. Issitt *The Challenge of Competence: Vocationalism through Education and Training*, London: Cassell.

——(1996) 'Competence in the quasi-market: towards the development of a feminist critique', Social Exclusion Research Monograph, Staffordshire University.

——(1999) 'Conceptualizing competence and reflective practice: a feminist perspective', in L. Cunningham, D. O'Reilly and S. Lester (eds), *Developing the capable practitioner through higher education*, London: Kogan Page.

Issitt, M. and Woodward, M. (1992) 'Competence and contradiction', in P. Carter, T. Jeffs and M.K. Smith (eds), *Changing Social Work and Welfare*, Buckingham: Open University Press.

Jones, L. and Moore, R. (1995) 'Appropriating competence: the competency movement, the New Right and the "culture change" project' *British Journal of Education and Work*, 8(2), 78–92.

Jordan, B. and Arnold, J. (1995) 'Democracy and criminal justice', *Critical Social Policy*, 15(2/3), 44/45, 170–82.

Knowles, M. (1986) *The Adult Learner – A Neglected Species*, Houston, Texas: Gulf Publishing. Cited in K. Ecclestone, 'The reflective practitioner: mantra or model for emancipation?' *Studies in the Education of Adults* 28(2),146–61.

Langan, M. and Day, L. (eds) (1992) *Women, Oppression and Social Work*, London: Routledge.

McNay, M. (1992) 'Social work and power relations: towards a framework for an integrated practice', in M. Langan and L. Day (eds), *Women, Oppression and Social Work* London: Routledge.

Martin, R. and Webster, G. (eds) (1994) *Women in Community Work: Feminist/Womanist Perspectives*, Sheffield: Federation of Community Work Training Groups.

Palmer, A., Burns, S. and Bulman, C. (1994) *Reflective Practice in Nursing: The Growth of the Professional Practitioner*, Oxford: Blackwell.

Pascall, G. (1997) *Social Policy: A New Feminist Analysis*, London: Routledge.

Pietroni, M. (1995) 'The nature and aims of professional education for social workers: a postmodern perspective', in M. Yelloly and M. Henkel (eds), *Learning and Teaching in Social Work: Towards Reflective Practice*, London: Jessica Kingsley.

Rogers, C. (1978) *On Personal Power*, London: Constable.

Schon, D. (1983) *The Reflective Practitioner*, New York: Basic Books.

——(1992) 'The crisis of professional knowledge and the pursuit of an epistemology of practice' *Journal of Interprofessional Care*, 6(1), 49–63.

Spicker, P. (1995) *Social Policy: Themes and Approaches*, Hemel Hempstead: Harvester Wheatsheaf.

Stanley, L. and Wise, S. (1993) *Breaking Out Again*, London: Routledge.

Thompson, N. (1995) *Theory and Practice in Health and Social Welfare*, Buckingham: Open University.

Tsang, N.M. (1998) 'Re-examining reflection – a common issue of professional concern in social work, teacher and nurse education', *Journal of Interprofessional Care*, 12(1), 21–31.

Walker, A. (1992) *In Search of Our Mothers' Gardens: Womanist Prose*, London: The Women's Press.

Williams, F. (1989) *Social Policy: A Critical Introduction*, Cambridge: Polity Press.

——(1996) 'Postmodernism, feminism and the question of difference', in N. Parton (ed.) *Social Theory, Social Change and Social Work*, London: Routledge.

Yelloly, M. and Henkel, M. (eds) (1995) *Learning and Teaching in Social Work: Towards Reflective Practice*, London: Jessica Kingsley.

Zeichner, K. (1994) 'Conceptions of reflective practice in teaching and teacher education', in G. Harvard and P. Hodkinson (eds), *Action and Reflection in Teacher Education*, New Jersey: Ablex.

8 Socio-economic factors

A neglected dimension in harm to children

Vic Tuck

This chapter argues that while physical abuse and neglect of children is likely to be influenced by many factors, more emphasis needs to be placed upon the socio-economic context in which parenting is performed and the possible consequences of this for children. Elsewhere I have reviewed evidence for the presence of complex inter-connections between poverty and the abuse of children (Tuck, forthcoming). Here I develop a framework for fuller understanding of the nature of these links, particularly how social deprivation contributes to situations where some parents physically injure or neglect their children. I aim to shed light on some of the pathways and processes that may in some circumstances lead to harmful outcomes for children. I shall argue that is it possible to develop multi-layered, multi-dimensional models which seek to account for links between social deprivation and harm to children, through examining interconnections between the practical resources available to parents, their social relationships and neighbourhood support networks. Such models do not minimize the importance of the personal characteristics and backgrounds of parents. These factors and others including the ability of individuals to cope with stress, the meanings they attribute to their experiences, and how they see themselves as coping with adversity, are likely to be important dimensions in these models. However, the argument in this chapter is that harm to children is powerfully linked to 'deficits' in material resources available to families and complex interacting psychosocial stress factors.

This needs to be seen in the context of a major increase in poverty in the UK over the last twenty years, and the growth of social inequalities (Goodman *et al.* 1997). The latter was confirmed in a study I undertook to compare the socio-economic characteristics of different neighbourhoods (Tuck 1995). More and more children are living in conditions of social disadvantage, leaving many poor parents experiencing a sense of social exclusion and abandonment, for which they perceive themselves to be held responsible by the wider society. An emphasis on the role of 'psychological stress factors' could be seen as compounding the perception of the poor as a deeply pathological social grouping, an 'underclass' in which children are treated in uniquely neglectful and violent ways. The political assaults on lone parent (female-headed) families are testimony to the dangers of such thinking.

This analysis does not see abuse of children as confined to socially disadvantaged people. Harm to children is present in all social classes (Pelton 1981). However, the presence of chronic multiple interacting deprivations, which characterizes the existence of the poorest families, may in some circumstances contribute to particularly stressful living conditions for children. It is these processes that this chapter endeavours to describe.

Social deprivation as a 'primary' and 'secondary' source of harm to children

In a study of adversities encountered by a group of mothers attempting to raise their children in a neighbourhood characterized by social disadvantage and high rates of child protection referrals to the local social services department, I found evidence to indicate that social deprivation represents both a primary and a secondary source of harm to children (Tuck 1995).

By imposing severe material constraints and environmental hazards on families, social deprivation limits the possibilities open to parents to care for their children safely and in good health. As such, it contributes to a situation of a general prevalence of harm. This is because socially disadvantaged families are likely to live in socially and economically impoverished neighbourhoods where it is difficult to maintain a healthy environment for children. Moreover, in contributing to social, material, interpersonal and intrapersonal barriers in families, social deprivation can prevent parents from achieving the standards of parenting they desire. The women in my study had clear views about the needs of their children, similar to the expectations of more affluent parents. But they confirmed Blackburn's (1991) research of poor parents constantly faced with difficult and often painful choices about which needs (including their own) will be met and which will go unmet. Sometimes there is no choice at all. For example, the women in my study identified the experience of being 'cooped up' with children in cramped, often unhealthy accommodation, as a major cause of stress and consequent harm to them. There was little scope to allow boisterous children to 'let off steam'. To allow them outside to play meant exposing them to unsuitable play areas in an unsafe environment. Neighbours would complain about noise and disruption. Faced with this, mothers generally kept their children at home (often only accessible by climbing numerous stairs) where pressures and tensions mounted.

In more affluent homes the choices available to families, including play-space and proper amenities, are more likely to be wider and more positive. For poor families choices are often about weighing up a series of unpromising options and selecting the least disadvantageous.

Aside from my study, there is a huge amount of research, back to studies of 'transmitted deprivation' in the 1970s and early 1980s, which highlight the deleterious impact of poverty and social deprivation on the health, safety and development of children – what I have termed as a *primary* source of harm. (For a review of these studies, see Blaxter 1993.)

However, parents who face chronic difficulties in meeting the basic needs of children may find that while this experience is likely to be undermining in itself, its consequences may in some situations be more serious still. The cumulative effects of coping with poor housing, low income, inadequate services and amenities for families, limited social support and social isolation, poor health and unsympathetic responses from some health professionals, and a sense of wider social abandonment, may contribute to circumstances where some parents may experience an acute sense of physical, psychological and emotional depletion. As the effects of these accumulate, the likelihood increases of high levels of psychosocial stress within families. In response to what may become intolerable pressures, some parents may experience a downward spiral of stress, inability to cope, helplessness and despair. This may manifest itself in harmful, destructive and punitive behaviours directed at their children. In these ways, social deprivation may come to constitute a *secondary* source of harm to children.

The complexities of these processes and the potential for multifarious outcomes, of which the physical abuse and neglect of children may be one set, should not be underestimated. A rigorous analysis of social deprivation as a potential secondary source of harm is needed. In my study, I sought to do this by interpreting the experiences and perceptions of the mothers who participated using a 'blend' of insights from sociological and psychological theory. The main elements in this 'blending' are concepts of psychosocial development (Rutter and others); studies of depression in women (Brown and Harris and others); theories of stress and stress reactions (Seligman and others); notions of 'learned helplessness' as elaborated by the same researcher and applied to social work by Barbar. Also included is 'social labelling' theory and its impact on people who feel themselves to be oppressed, marginalized and stigmatized by the wider society. Underpinning this attempt to develop interpretative frameworks based on a number of perspectives is an 'interactionist–social constructionist' approach as applied to the impact of social deprivation on human functioning, especially the perceptions which individuals come to hold of themselves and their ability to cope in the face of adversity.

The way this material is synthesized for the purposes of my analysis may run contrary to the intentions of the original authors, but this does not diminish their usefulness to the concerns of this chapter.

Psychosocial development, social deprivation and harm to children

> Plenty of people would rather declare an event incredible than follow the sequence of cause and effect, measure the strength of links in a chain, each arising from the one before it and inseverably joined with it, secretly, in the mind.
>
> (de Balzac *et al.*, quoted in Brown 1988: 285)

In quoting de Balzac, Brown argues for greater attention to be paid to the importance of causal paths, chains and strands in human development. Accordingly, I reflect on some key themes in theories of psychosocial risk and development, setting this against some of the implications for children and families living in social disadvantage. From there I develop propositions about possible interactions between social deprivation, psychosocial stress and harm to children, and describe a possible process that may shed light on these interactions.

Five main threads will run through the analysis:

- risk prediction based upon the identification-a single or several variables at specific times cannot account for the complexity of causal paths leading to child abuse (Baldwin and Spencer 1993);
- causal relationships need instead to be examined in the form of chains and linked sequences involving several different and short-term effects (Rutter 1988);

- the chains of events at work are likely to be linked in different ways and in different orders to each individual or family (Blaxter 1993);
- these chains, sequences and relationships need to be understood within the socio-economic context in which they occur, recognizing the stress which poverty and deprivation can generate in families and communities;
- the outcomes they give rise to are likely to be influenced by the 'meanings' which individuals attribute to their experiences and actions, and how they come to perceive themselves.

This last thread confirms how the analysis presented here is influenced by a 'cognitive–social constructionist' perspective of human behaviour and response.

Risk and protective factors

The study of psychosocial development has been concerned with the way 'risk' and 'protective' factors influence outcomes, and how and when these variables operate at different points in the life-span (Kolvin *et al.* 1988). As the interactionist perspective advanced by both Brown (1988) and Rutter (1988) suggests, a focus on the 'person-process-context paradigm' can be helpful in conceptualizing strategies for managing risk and protective factors in psychosocial development (Rainer *et al.* 1988).

Rutter has defined 'protective factors' as those influences 'that modify, ameliorate or alter a person's response to some environmental hazard that predisposes to a maladaptive outcome' (Rutter 1985: 600).

'Risk' may be considered both in terms of experience and of an individual's reaction to experience. It is: 'a dynamic concept varying within individuals according to their circumstances and their reactions to an event will depend on these factors and on their stock of previous experience and of the temperament that they have to contend with experience' (Wadsworth 1988: 256).

Wadsworth refers to the importance of the individual's 'circumstances' as a risk variable. We can view 'circumstances' in a relatively narrow light – histories and personal characteristics of individuals only – or it can encompass the socio-economic context in which individuals and families function. A narrow interpretation would reflect the concerns of those who have applied a 'family pathology' or 'family dysfunction' perspective to the study of harm to children (cf. Browne *et al.* 1988; Dale *et al.* 1986). However, harm to children is a highly

complex interactional process. Individual factors are in constant interplay, not only with factors in the immediate family environment but
also with those associated with the socio-economic circumstances of
children and parents (the material and practical resources to which
families have access and the quality of the neighbourhoods where they
live). These will enhance or constrain the opportunities for safe and
healthy development available to them.

'Environment' is a problematic term. Does it refer solely to the
immediate circumstances of individuals and families or does it also
embrace wider social structural contexts and the impact of social
inequalities on people? In this discussion, these wider definitions are
applied and the concepts of psychosocial development are extended
into broader terrain.

Resilience and coping

The interplay of 'resilience' and 'coping' has also been a concern of
theories about psychosocial development: 'Many potentially adverse
life events occur apparently by chance; in the face of an adverse experience the individual degree of vulnerability or invulnerability depends
on the nature of coping or reacting' (Wadsworth 1988: 256).

These two factors are associated with the individual's attributes and
previous experience. Moreover, life experiences vary in their risk potential. Rutter argues that throughout life it is normal to meet challenges
and overcome difficulties. Coping successfully with stress situations
can be strengthening: 'The promotion of resilience does not lie in the
avoidance of stress, but rather in encountering stress at a time and in a
way that allows self-confidence and social competence to increase
through mastery and appropriate responsibility' (Rutter 1985: 608).

Equally, protection does not lie in the 'buffering effect' of one
supportive factor which operates at one point in time. The quality of
resilience rests in part upon how people deal with life changes and
what they do about their situations. This is likely to be influenced by
experiences in early life, childhood and adolescence, and by circumstances in adult life: 'None of these is in itself determinate of later
outcomes, but in combination they may serve to create a chain of indi-
rect linkages that foster [or deny] escape from adversity' (Rutter 1985:
608).

Crucially, resistance to stress is relative rather than absolute. The
basis of resistance is both environmental and constitutional: the degree
of resistance will vary over time and according to circumstance. To
take this further, the degree of resistance may be influenced by many

possible and changing interacting factors including personal history and characteristics, the practical resources available, and social relationships and support networks. Here another factor in psychosocial development becomes vital.

Interactive processes

In his study of children facing chronic adversities (e.g. parental discord, mental disorder, overcrowding), Rutter found that no one of these had any effect on psychiatric risk when it occurred in isolation. The psychiatric risk rose sharply when several adversities co-existed (Rutter 1979). He reached similar conclusions in a study of children with repeated hospital admissions who experienced a high degree of psychosocial adversity in their family circumstances (Quinton and Rutter 1976). For them, the likelihood of experiencing emotional disturbance was greater than for those experiencing hospital admissions alone. Rutter (1981) accounts for this in terms of adverse effects potentiating one another so that their combined effects become greater than the sum of the two considered separately.

This has implications for an assessment of the interplay between psychosocial risk, social deprivation and harm to children. But first it is necessary to consider in more detail some of the implications of social disadvantage for children and families.

Continuities of disadvantage and harm to children

Kolvin *et al.* (1988) have studied the links between juvenile offending and social deprivation. They demonstrate how the more deprivations there are co-existing in families, the higher the rate of subsequent offending by boys. Families who move out of deprivation tend to be characterized by a significant decrease in the rate of offending. Those who move *into* deprivation face an equally significant increase in the rate of offending. The movement out of deprivation seemed to give some protection in families, while movement into deprivation increased vulnerability.

A similar process may operate in relation to harm to children. Where a cluster of adversities, including those generated by social deprivation, are experienced in families, then the vulnerability of children to harm may be heightened. Where these are ameliorated and the continuity of deprivation broken, families may experience greater protection, reducing the risk of harm to children. In my study, the experience of all the families was one of facing numerous adversities and hindrances to good parenting. Two of the women interviewed who admitted to having injured their children were clear that it was this accumulation of adversity and stress that had played a decisive part in the harmful outcomes to the children. When services were provided that offset the pressures faced by them, they described how parenting became less difficult and the children were at less risk of direct harm.

In tackling child abuse and neglect, this suggests that if we are to be more effective in preventing physical injury, an objective of service provision for families should be the interruption of continuities of disadvantage which may interact with other factors to heighten risks. It implies the strengthening of 'protective factors' which may exist within families and communities. This is similar to recent research findings commissioned by central government in the UK (Department of Health, 1995). I return to this later.

However, again it is important not to underestimate the complexities of these situations. Account needs to be taken of other factors that influence the degree of risk. I shall consider three of these briefly.

Possible long-term effects of social deprivation on children and families

Essen and Wedge (1982) found that multiple disadvantage at any age is likely to have long-term damaging consequences for life chances of children. They discovered apparent continuing developmental delay in many young people even if they are no longer disadvantaged. Moving out of social deprivation, therefore, may not in itself mean that children will no longer experience negative and harmful outcomes. It is possible that the degree of risk may be diminished but some risk, whether a damaging developmental outcome or more direct risk of harm, may still remain. Schorr (1988) has also argued that multiple disadvantage is likely to be sufficiently destructive to guarantee the persistent presence of a collection of psychosocial risk factors over a long period of time.

Personal characteristics and background of parents

There is some evidence then, of the continuing destructive impact of poverty and social deprivation. Another factor influencing the risk of harm may be the personal strengths and limitations of parents in coping with adversity. Rutter (1985) has argued that a person's ability to act positively and to resist adversity is a function of their self-esteem, feelings of efficacy and problem-solving skills. Their ability to develop a positive 'cognitive set' to mobilize coping strategies and adaptive behaviours is likely to be influenced by such varied features as secure and stable affectional relationships; success and achievement; ability to appraise experiences, attach 'meaning' to them and integrate them into their stock of experience. Another feature is likely to be the interaction over time of personal qualities in response to others.

Whether these features have a strengthening effect which promotes resilience will be influenced by complex chains of events and linked sequences involving several different and short-term effects (Rutter 1988). These chains of events are likely to be linked in different ways and in different orders in different individuals and families (Blaxter 1993). Moving in and out of social deprivation, experiencing disadvantage intermittently or remaining in disadvantage indefinitely (the experience of the families in my study) is one aspect of these sequences.

What are the consequences of these personal features as they interact with the experience of social deprivation? Fisher (1984) has postulated that someone who feels in control of events may be able to cope more effectively with stress than a person who does not feel in control. The importance of a positive 'cognitive set' is that it helps equip a person with this sense of control. However, social deprivation may weaken a person's belief that they can exercise control. The frequent experience of reduced control may compound feelings that control is rarely possible in life, increasing pessimism about one's ability to solve problems. As Rutter observes, 'what is characteristic of so many people who experience chronic stress and adversity is that they feel helpless to do anything about their life situation' (1985: 607).

Barbar (1986), in an appraisal of 'learned helplessness' theory and its applications to social work, argues that its value lies in its articulation of a psychology of powerlessness. It can provide an insight into the world of the poor and the oppressed: people who are regularly confronted by events beyond their control. For people living in social deprivation, choice is limited and control over 'valued outcomes' resides elsewhere. An expectation may develop that responding and outcome are independent of one another, and this effect comes to be characterized by its capacity to generalize beyond the situation in which it originally developed. A more general sense of 'uncontrollability', as Seligman (1975, 1978) has observed, may then give rise to resignation and despair.

It can be argued that some parents facing the chronic debilitating effects of exposure to social deprivation may succumb to 'learned helplessness' as they perceive their efforts to 'keep their heads above water' as unsuccessful: 'nothing I do seems to help', 'things are getting worse', 'everything is out of control'. The sense of resignation, despair and frustration to which such attributions of meaning may give rise could spell dangers for some children. Combinations of these feelings and cognition could manifest themselves in parental indifference or neglect, or in violent reactions towards children, triggered at times of extreme personal and familial stress. It is then that a cycle of cumulative harm may result as parents find themselves locked into resignation and despair – a continual undermining of their sense of self-efficacy from which it becomes difficult to demonstrate adaptive behaviours again.

There was some evidence of this in the lives of the mothers in my study. Yet for most it did not result in the passivity in the face of life events that Barbar observes as a major feature of 'learned helplessness'. On the contrary, most battled in the face of enormous odds, and even those who did injure their children were able to regain some control eventually, overcoming their sense of resignation and despair enough to care safely again for their children. This may in part be accounted for by a third factor influencing the degree of risk experienced by children in families.

Balancing psychosocial stress and social support in families

In two studies, Rutter found that even in the face of the most acute stress and adversity, people generally demonstrate substantial resilience. For example, the risk of depression following disturbing life events might well be increased, but most people do not become depressed (Rutter 1985). One reason for this could lie not just in the strength or otherwise of a person's 'cognitive set', but also in the interplay of 'vulnerability factors', 'provoking agents' (Brown and Harris 1978, Brown *et al.* 1987) and 'buffering influences' (Rutter 1985) – the operation of, on the one hand, factors and agents that increase a person's susceptibility to 'stressors' and, on the other hand, influences such as the level of social support enjoyed by an individual or family, performing a 'protective' function. Brown and Harris, in their studies of women experiencing depression, define vulnerability factors as absence of a close confiding relationship, the presence of young children, social isolation, lack of self-esteem and feelings of lack of control. Key provoking agents of depression in women were separation or threat of separation from a key figure through death or serious illness, major material loss, loss of employment or a failure to attain personal goals.

Significantly, Brown and Harris identified a major social class component in this experience. Rates of depression were significantly higher among working-class women with children than among comparable middle-class women. Working-class women are more likely to suffer more severe difficulties involving social loss. Blackburn (1991) notes that, with the exception of losing one's mother before the age of 11, the vulnerability factors identified by Brown and Harris are all linked to the women's socio-economic position. Blackburn accounts for this in terms of living on low income, which is likely to determine social class experience: 'Material loss and social loss have greater implications for low-income families, particularly women in low-income families' (Blackburn 1991: 111).

As my study confirms, this is because women bear the brunt of poverty. They are the 'gatekeepers' of family health and, as chief care-givers, frequently experience the worry and stress of budgeting to make ends meet, and managing debts. Working-class women, therefore, feel acutely the lack of cushioning against social loss which higher income and good living conditions provide (Blackburn 1991: 111).

However, the interplay of vulnerability factors and provoking agents is likely to be influenced by the degree of social support experienced by parents, particularly mothers as chief care-givers. Positive relationships with partners, relatives, friends and neighbours have a protective effect against stressful life events and circumstances. These relationships may enhance feelings of self-esteem and self-efficacy and offer a strengthened basis of emotional and practical support.

Chamberlin (1988) argues that, for children and families, the ability to provide a healthy environment is strongly related to their ability to cope with the balance between stress, their coping capacities and social support. Parental perceptions of their own success in dealing with adversity are also likely to be important influences in managing this balance. Where stressors accumulate to outweigh protective factors in a family's circumstances, this balance may tip towards negative outcomes for children. Thus, harm to children may be influenced by problems individuals and families face in maintaining some equilibrium between stress, coping and support.

Again, the complexities should not be underestimated. The mix of interrelated variables that may come into play over time – movements in and out of social disadvantage (there may be no such movements for some families), psychological resources of parents, the interplay of vulnerability factors, provoking agents, buffering influences, the characteristics and behaviour of the children themselves – these and other factors make it difficult to predict which individuals and families will 'tip over' into harmful outcomes for their children.

However, on the basis of this 'blending' of theoretical insights and concepts, supported to some extent by research, it is possible to identify pathways which may shed light on the possible connections between social deprivation and harm to children. The following models are informed by 'interactionist' (cf. Plummer 1983) and 'social constructionist' perspectives (cf. Gergen 1982, 1985; Bluner 1990), which emphasize the role of 'social actors' and the meanings they attribute to their experiences and actions. Therefore I define this model as a 'cognitive–social constructionist' model of harm to children.

A cognitive–social constructionist model of harm to children

Figure 8.1 describes the model diagrammatically.

In this model, psychosocial stress is defined according to three categories which, as sources of stress, are likely to link together and interact:

1 The *neighbourhood* in which social-disadvantaged families live – where they are likely to encounter a range of adversities such as poor housing, poor social amenities and a generally poor-quality social environment characterized by high levels of crime, vandalism, a prevailing sense of 'unsafeness' and a range of other social problems. These families, as in my study, are likely to have low incomes, feel themselves to be poorly supported and isolated – social support networks may be inadequate – and may experience poor health. These adversities may prevent parents from achieving the standards of parenting they would like.

2 *Individual and family factors* such as the personal history and characteristics of parents, the 'cognitive set' they have developed in response to life events, the behavioural and emotional characteristics of children, and family relationships. The material resources and social supports available to individuals and families will also be important. There are likely to be many more factors with the potential to contribute to stress.

3 *External attributions*: negative public and professional perceptions of the neighbourhood and its inhabitants. Here, stress arises from the sense of stigmatization of such labels, and the reinforcement of negative self-perceptions. It is also linked to the influence of 'ruling ideas' about what constitutes 'good parenting' and how

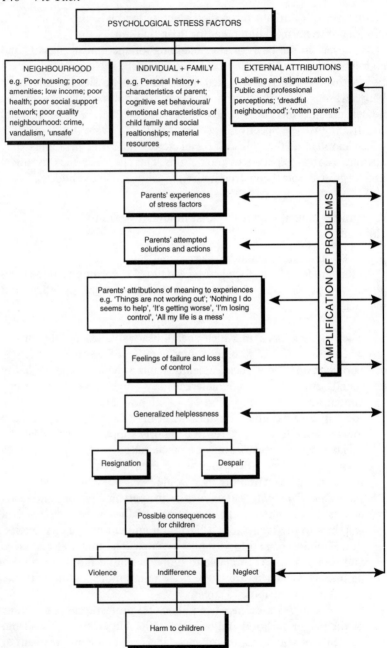

Figure 8.1   Cognitive–social constructivist model of harm to children

individuals are likely to perceive themselves if they are seen and feel themselves to be failing to meet these socially constructed expectations. These issues emerged in my study as powerful influences in the lives of the mothers and their families, and it was useful to apply concepts associated with social labelling theory to interpret their experiences and perceptions (cf. Bilton *et al.* 1987).

The major implication of the labelling process rests on the assumption that a 'deviant' label, which is how socially deprived parents living in 'rough' neighbourhoods may be seen by the wider public and social agencies, has important effects on how people may come to regard themselves and on the subsequent patterns of interactions between them and others. This is because the ascription of deviant status results in individual actors and the social group around them accommodating themselves to a 'spoiled identity'. This in turn has consequences for the individual's further social participation and self-image. A process of stigmatization occurs where one's public identity is re-evaluated as one is labelled as a certain 'kind' of person. The mothers in my study described how they thought the wider world saw them, indicating the possible operation of these processes: 'They [outsiders] see us as slags'; 'They think we're just a bunch of rough-necks who can't look after their children properly'; 'You can see people's faces change when you tell them where you live'.

In response to experiences of these and other factors, parents may try to alleviate stress by attempting to find solutions to the problems. On the basis of the actions and the degree of success they yield or are perceived to yield, parents will continue to attribute 'meanings' to their actions and experiences. If these actions are felt to be unsuccessful, or if individuals feel that the demands being made upon them are simply beyond their capacity to manage, then this may lead to feelings of failure and a perception that control of one's life is being lost. The cumulative effect of this, particularly if they are reinforced by negative external attributions, may be a more generalized sense of helplessness leading to resignation and despair on the part of the parent. If these feelings and perceptions are not alleviated, such as might happen where there are relatively strong support systems, and problems continue to escalate, then in some situations this could result in indifferent, neglectful or violent responses towards children.

The systemic nature of this model highlights how these situations can become a vicious circle. At various points in the process, the negative feelings and cognitions experienced by socially disadvantaged parents may be amplified by the attributions attached to their experiences, actions and coping capacities by the surrounding society. The stigmatization which flows from being labelled as 'useless', unable to cope and as inadequate parents may compound the feelings of failure and loss of control already felt by parents struggling against the odds to care adequately for their children. Thus the cycle may be perpetuated with even more serious consequences for children and families.

Limitations and implications

In this chapter I have sought to map out an account of how links between social deprivation and harm to children may operate, and some possible outcomes. I have acknowledged throughout the presentation of this 'integrative' model (based on a blending of sociological and psychological theory) that there are likely to be many more factors to consider than I have been able to address here. For example, it is necessary to understand how these processes and pathways are likely to be mediated by the racial, religious and cultural backgrounds of individuals and families, and by disability. My study focused on the experiences of a small group of women. Women are likely to be the chief care-givers, and there is a need to explore far more how the gender of parents will impact upon and shape the processes I have described. Even in situations of physical injury it is still predominantly men who cause direct harm to children (Parton 1990). Moreover, caution needs to be exercised in applying these models to sexual abuse, where yet more complex factors come into play.

Nevertheless, by mapping out terrain which may deepen our understanding of some aspects of the aetiology of child abuse and linking this to social divisions arising from the status of parents (especially working-class female single parents) it is possible to draw conclusions about the types of services and strategies which families, particularly those who are socially disadvantaged, need to raise their children safely. This analysis may also contribute to our understanding of how 'welfare' itself may be developed to resist the patterns of social divisions which have been the concern of this chapter.

The processes and models I have outlined point to the importance of interventive strategies which have as their major focus the needs of 'vulnerable' populations of children and families rather than attempting exclusively to identify individual families where harm to children might be occurring. Within populations of socially disadvantaged families, there may be any number of parents who could succumb to the processes described here and eventually present to social agencies as 'high risk' cases. We cannot tell with any accuracy who will 'tip over' into producing a harmful outcome for their children. The challenge to social welfare agencies is to recognize and respond to the link between stress, coping capacities and support. As Chamberlin (1988) has observed, once a family has moved from the 'medium risk' status that is likely to characterize most of those families living in areas with high exposure to psychosocial stress factors, into a 'high risk' status, then it becomes much more difficult to retrieve the situation. Chamberlin argues for movement beyond the confines of 'individual risk assessment' towards community-wide approaches which have a much sharper child welfare focus and are based on the provision of comprehensive and co-ordinated family welfare services. These arguments rest well with much current thinking on the balance to be struck between child protection and family support (Department of Health 1995).

They also 'fit' with arguments advanced by Abramson *et al.* (1978) that in order to alleviate the effects of learned helplessness syndrome it is necessary to promote 'environmental enrichment' where attempts are made to reverse the expectation that responding is useless. The provision of services that offer a range of practical and emotional support to families may help to ameliorate the helplessness 'deficits' that tend to characterize this condition and assist parents to recognize that valued outcomes can be achieved. This is not to say that some individuals and families may not be so depleted by their experiences of social disadvantage, an experience shared by perhaps many generations of their family, that considerable levels of support may be needed before any improvement is experienced, and even then there is no guarantee of this. There may also be more complex factors at work, requiring interventions at an interpersonal, intrapersonal and familial level as well as the broader strategies outlined here. Ultimately, however, enhancing parents' coping capacities in this way could strengthen their ability to provide a safer healthier environment for their children.

An objective of a genuinely progressive approach to welfare in the UK, as the new millennium approaches, can be the development of means by which continuities of disadvantage can be interrupted, as indicated earlier in this chapter. The provision of comprehensive co-ordinated multi-agency services for families living in areas of high social need will not eliminate these continuities – this will require, as it always has done, major long-term shifts in social and economic policy aimed at tackling social inequalities. However, refocusing provision to recognize the daily realities of life for the families it is meant to assist, seeking to counter the deleterious effects of those realities, may open up fresh prospects for welfare.

Conclusion

What of the implications of these models for the critical professional in the contemporary context? Social workers have tended to make sense of their clients' experiences predominantly through traditional psychological models of human development. This has resulted in the pathologizing of particular groups of families, particularly working-class families. This has been compounded by images of single parents (largely women) as inadequate and as largely to blame for their situation. The 'underclass' (Murray 1994) is imagined as the depository of those who exist on the fringes of society, neglecting and abusing their children. An implication of the models I have described here is that there needs to be a serious recognition of the part played by poverty, with its massive injustices and inequalities, and its destruction of well-being and spirit. Poverty affects not a minority but a substantial part of the population, with almost two-thirds living below the average income level (Novak 1996), and as I have argued, poverty exists along-side wider evidences of social deprivation. If these are significant factors in parental abuse of children, then they should be a priority for government policy.

At the same time, if personal strengths and social supports are also important, critical professionals will need to recognize, build on and work with these resources within poor communities. The parents in my study found themselves under great strain which sometimes resulted in harm to their children. They also showed strengths in organization, and in budgeting, and had aspirations for themselves and their children. Social workers need to find ways of working with these ambitions, alongside both individuals and their social supports. Listening to the needs and perceptions of families and communities, and taking what is heard seriously, lies at the heart of an 'interactionist–social constructionist' model. It requires that professionals, policy-makers and service providers at all levels endeavour to understand the meanings that are attributed to events, circumstances and conditions by those on the receiving end. How do they define the difficulties they face? How do they view the solutions to those difficulties? What do they see themselves as needing if they are to manage their lives, look after themselves and those in their care? What are their strengths, and how can they be built upon?

Inevitably there will be tensions and conflicts because perceptions will differ. Sometimes the needs of the child, at risk of harm, may come before those of other people. But the whole process of assessing human needs and the risks faced by vulnerable people should be based on openness, negotiation and partnership where the objective is to empower rather than compound a sense of helplessness, resignation and despair.

Such an approach is not just applicable to interactions between professionals, individuals and families. It should inform the processes of strategic planning, delivery and review of services in local areas. Agencies can work more closely with local communities to help them empower themselves, rather than imposing the corporate view of things. In this way it may also become possible for social agencies to respond more effectively to difference and diversity in populations.

The part played by poverty and social deprivation in neglect and harm to children has been played down, even made invisible, in the models adopted to explain the abuse of children. Of course, it is not the only factor, as I have tried to show, but it needs to be exposed as a start in bringing pressure on government to do something about its causes.

References

Abramson, L.Y., Seligman, M.E.P. and Teasdale, J.D. (1978) 'Learned helplessness in humans: critique and reformulation', *Journal of Abnormal Psychology*, 87, 49–74.

Baldwin, N. and Spencer, N. (1993) 'Deprivation and child abuse: implications for strategic planning in children's services', *Children and Society*, 7 (4), 277–96.

Barbar, J.C. (1986) 'The promise and pitfalls of learned helplessness theory for social work practice', *British Journal of Social Work*, 16, 570–7.

Bilton, T., Bonnet, K., Jones, P., Stanworth, M., Sheard, K. and Webster, A. (1987) *Introductory Sociology* (second edition), London: Macmillan Education.

Blackburn, C. (1991) *Poverty and Health: Working with Families*, Milton Keynes: Open University Press.

Blaxter, M. (1993) *Continuities of Disadvantage and Child Health*, Andover: Intercept.

Bluner, J. (1990) *Acts of Meaning*, New York: Harvard University Press.

Brown, B.W., Bifulco, A. and Harris, T.O. (1987) 'Life events, vulnerability and onset of depression: some late refinements', *British Journal of Psychiatry*, 150, 30–42.

Brown, G.W. (1988) 'Causal paths, chains and strains', in M. Rutter (ed.), *Studies of Psychosocial Risk: The Power of Longitudinal Data*, Cambridge: Cambridge University Press.

Brown, G.W. and Harris, T.O. (1978) *The Social Origins of Depression*, London: Tavistock.

152   *Vic Tuck*

Browne, K., Davies, C. and Stratton, P. (eds) (1988) *Early Prediction and Prevention of Child Abuse*, Chichester: Wiley.

Chamberlin, R.W. (ed.) (1988) *Beyond Individual Risk Assessment: Community-wide Approaches to Promoting the Health and Development of Families and Children*, in the edited and expanded version of the Proceedings of a Conference Held in Hanover, New Hampshire, 1–4 November 1987, Washington DC: The Maternal and Child Health Clearing House.

Dale, P., Davies, M., Morrison, T. and Waters, J. (1986) *Dangerous Families: Assessment and the Treatment of Child Abuse*, London: Tavistock.

Department of Health (1995) *Child Protection: Messages from Research*, London: HMSO.

Essen, J. and Wedge, P. (1982) *Continuities in Childhood Disadvantage*, London: Heinemann Educational Books.

Fisher, S. (1984) *Stress and the Perception of Control*, London: Lawrence Earlbaum Associates.

Gergen, K.J. (1982) *Towards Transformation in Social Knowledge*, New York: Springer-Verlay.

——(1985) 'The social constructionist movement in modern psychology', *American Psychologist*, 40 (3), 266–75.

Goodman, A., Johnson, P. and Webb, S. (1997) *Inequality in the UK*, Oxford, New York: Oxford University Press.

Kolvin, I., Miller, F.J.W., Fleeting, M. and Kolvin, P.A. (1988) 'Risk, protective factors for offending with particular reference to deprivation', in M. Rutter (ed.), *Studies of Psychosocial Risk: The Power of Longitudinal Data*, Cambridge: Cambridge University Press.

Murray, C. (1994) *Underclass: The Crisis Deepens*, London: IEA Health and Welfare Unit, Choice in Welfare Series, no. 20.

Novak, T. (1996) 'Empowerment and the Politics of Poverty', in B. Humphries (ed.), *Critical Perspectives on Empowerment*, Birmingham: Venture Press, 85–98.

Parton, C. (1990) 'Women, gender oppression and child abuse', in The Violence Against Children Study Group, *Taking Child Abuse Seriously: Contemporary Issues in Child Protection Theory and Practice*, London: Unwin Hyman.

Pelton, L. (1981) 'The myth of classlessness', in L. Pelton (ed.), *The Social Context of Child Abuse and Neglect*, London: Human Sciences Press.

Plummer, K. (1983) *Documents of Life: An Introduction to the Problems and Literature of Humanistic Method*, London: Unwin Hyman.

Quinton, D. and Rutter, M. (1976) 'Early hospital admissions and later disturbance of behaviour: an attempted replication of Douglas's findings', *Developmental Medicine Child Neurology*, 18, 441–59.

Rainer, K., Silbereisen, S. and Walper, S. (1988) 'A person-process-context approach', in M. Rutter (ed.), *Studies of Psychosocial Risk: The Power of Longitudinal Data*, Cambridge: Cambridge University Press.

Rutter, M. (1979) 'Protective factors in children's responses to stress and disadvantage', in M.W. Kent and J.E. Rolf (eds), *Primary Prevention of*

Psychopathology vol. 3: Social Competence in Children, New Hampshire: University Press of New England.

——(1981) 'Stress, coping and developing: some issues and some perspectives', *Journal of Child Psychology and Psychiatry*, 22, 322–56.

——(1985) 'Resilience in the face of adversity: protective factors and resistance to psychiatric disorder', *British Journal of Psychiatry*, 147, 598–611.

Rutter, M. (ed.) (1988) *Studies of Psychosocial Risk: The Power of Longitudinal Data*, Cambridge: Cambridge University Press.

Schorr, L.B. (1988) *Within Our Reach: Breaking the Cycle of Disadvantage*, Doubleday.

Seligman, M.E. (1975) *Helplessness on Depression, Development and Death*, San Francisco: W.H. Freeman.

——(1978) 'Comment and integration', *Journal of Abnormal Psychology*, 87, 165–79.

Tuck, V. (1995) 'Links between social deprivation and harm to children: a study of parenting in social deprivation', unpublished PhD thesis, Open University.

—— (forthcoming) 'Links between social deprivation and harm to children', in N. Baldwin (ed.), *Protecting Children: Promoting Their Rights*, London: Whiting and Birch.

Wadsworth, M.E.J. (1988) 'Intergenerational longitudinal research: conceptual and methodological considerations', in M. Rutter (ed.), *Studies of Psychosocial Risk: The Power of Longitudinal Data*, Cambridge: Cambridge University Press.

9 School exclusion

Alienation and the dilemmas for formal and informal educators

Carol Packham

Introduction

Schools have always failed some young people. Their very nature and purpose results in the institutional exclusion of some and the self-exclusion of others who find the constraints of a controlling environment intolerable. This chapter explores the reasons for school exclusions and their apparent increase. It locates the rise in youth work involvement with schools, and suggests that some strategies are perpetuating, rather than preventing, pupils' alienation.

The view that 'excluded' pupils are disaffected implies that they have no will to participate and that they are problematic, non-conformist, unable or disabled. Explanations for exclusion have focused on problematizing the young person or their 'parents', or blaming poor teachers or teaching methods (OFSTED 1996; UNISON/NASWE 1998). This fails to recognize that schools have a responsibility to enable young people to engage with education in ways meaningful to them. The problematizing approach also fails to locate the school within an economic, political and social framework.

Several factors have coincided to make evident the failure of schools for many young people. Some exclusion has been systematic and disguised either by definition – for example, the segregation of disabled young people into 'special schools' – or by class, gender, sexuality and race assumptions of inferiority, limited potential and biological determinism (e.g. Eysenck 1970). This covert discrimination became apparent with the publication of the number of permanently excluded young people (January 1996 DoE) and the categorization of excluded young people by gender and ethnicity (DoE 1994/95). This revealed a substantial increase in exclusions and the high levels of exclusion of particular groups, e.g. boys of African-Caribbean origin – 0.66 per cent as compared to 0.18 per cent white (DoE 1996). While the concern over black under-achievement was voiced loudly by black groups (Osler 1997; Commission for Racial Equality 1997), the issue only became cause for general concern by being coupled with a purported increase in male under-achievement among all groups. It is quite possible that the matter of who was continuing to be 'excluded' would have remained uncontentious had the system for recording permanent exclusions not changed in September 1994 (Circular 10/94, DoE 1994). Prior to this, excluded pupils could be kept on school rolls indefinitely. The new system allowed the school to temporarily exclude for a maximum of 15 days in any one term, or permanently exclude. This new and restrictive system resulted in a dramatic rise in the numbers of young people being permanently excluded (from 2,910 in 1990–91 to 13,581 in 1996–7, in addition to the 100,000 temporary exclusions per year (Pearce and Hillman 1998: 1). This made public the pupils who were a cause for concern, and alerted people to the weakness of the educational system that was failing them.

Young people spend a total of 15,000 hours in school. It is therefore a 'major instrument of socialization in advanced industrialised societies' (Bilton 1994: 304). Young people alienated from this process are therefore seen as a threat, particularly if they do not take their exclusion passively. Anxieties regarding the excluded are fuelled by statistics which show that 65 per cent of school-age offenders sentenced in court have been excluded or truant significantly (Audit Commission 1996). The connection between exclusion and crime is further highlighted by the Social Exclusion Unit, who state that 'many of today's non-attenders are in danger of becoming tomorrow's criminals and unemployed' (1998: 1). Pearce and Hillman (1998) see these young people, and particularly young men, as being dehumanized and labelled as 'rat boys' and 'underwolves' by the press. Excluded boys are therefore perceived as becoming alienated men, a challenge to law and order, and a long-term risk to the harmony of society.

The alarm over school exclusions may abate as a result of the changes in the system of reporting permanent exclusions (1997 Education Act). Pupils can now be excluded for a total of 45 days in any one academic year, as opposed to 15 days in any one term previously. This gives more time to resolve issues, or to wait until a pupil is legally old enough to leave school. This gives the opportunity for a statistical manipulation of the problem reducing numbers of reported permanent exclusions, placating concern among schools about their positioning in 'league tables'. Such moves may only serve to disguise the failure of formal education for many young people. Here I shall argue that there have always been large groups of young people whose exclusion and under-achievement has gone, and will continue to go, unrecognized and unresolved unless the fundamental nature and structure of formal education is challenged. Employing youth work skills in formal education, particularly to 'deal' with excluded and 'disaffected' pupils, is increasingly popular. I will explore the dilemmas posed for youth workers and other educators who, while seeking to work in schools in a participatory way, have brought to the fore the clash between principles and methods for critical practitioners.

Explanations for school exclusion

The explanations for school exclusion can be classified into four main areas: those in relation to *policy*, i.e. the increasingly centralized and legal requirements placed on local delivery of education; *practice*, e.g. curriculum, methodology, relationships and ethos of schools; *personal*, or individual factors relating to the 'excluded' pupil; and *public*, or societal influences and attitudes that impinge on the pupils and their schools (see Figure 9.1). All of these elements ('blades' of the propeller on Figure 9.1) interrelate and should be considered when debating causes and strategies for tackling exclusion. For example, without change at the public, policy and practice levels there will always be individuals whose experience will be excluded from education. I shall discuss these factors in turn.

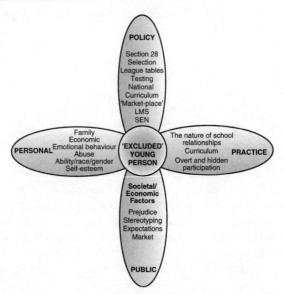

Figure 9.1   Exclusion propeller: factors attributing to exclusion

Policy

Policy is recognized as an important determinant of social behaviour. The Conservative Right as represented by Charles Murray (1990) suggests that a 'youth underclass' of excluded young people has emerged as a result of liberal welfare policies. Others blame the erosion of the welfare state and comprehensive provision of education for all as a cause of exclusion. For example, the 1988 Education Reform Act (ERA) has had far-reaching consequences on all involved with formal education and the opportunities available, in particular on young people alienated from school. Local authorities now have a reduced involvement with the management and financing of state schools, parents and community members being encouraged, by new rights of governance, to be involved in local management of schools. Parents have been given the right to chose schools for their children. However, choice is greatest for those with mobility and whose children are deemed desirable: for example, schools can refuse to admit young people who have been excluded twice (Schools Standards and Framework Bill 1997).

Formal education has become a competition-driven market-place, based on the publication of pupils' test results, absences and exclusions tables, and with reduced opportunities for teachers and pupils alike (Sanders and Hendry 1997). This has resulted in concentration on successful pupils (i.e. those obtaining grades A–C at GCSE) at the expense of a growing and significant minority of failing young people. For example, in 1997, 81,228 failed Maths, English and Combined Science GCSE compared with 113,121 in 1998 (Hart 1998).

The Social Exclusion Unit Report on Truancy and School Exclusion (1998) recognizes that the rise in exclusions could be attributed to 'reasons relating to educational climate and policy' (p. 11), citing the increased pressures faced by schools as a result of performance tables, reducing the willingness or ability to keep 'problematic' young people within school. These findings are further supported by research in Northern Ireland, which indicated a reduced tolerance for disruptive pupils resulting in a sharp rise in 'suspensions and expulsions'. This was felt to be contributed to by education reforms and schools trying to balance the business ethos with that of their professional standards (Kilpatrick and Barr 1997).

Schools' concentration on successful pupils has coincided with an increased ability to remove 'problematic' pupils. The *Pupils with Problems* Circulars 8–13 (DoE 1994) gave a new definition of 'education otherwise'. Prior to this, the term had been used in connection with 'alternative education' arrangements made as a positive *choice* to mainstream school. Education 'otherwise' enabled the establishment of 'pupil referral units' (Circular 11, DoE 1994), for excluded pupils, which were funded by the transfer of money allocated to schools for individual pupils (1993 Education Act and DoE Circular 19/94). These units were often off school premises and, although designed to reintegrate pupils back into mainstream school, tended to concentrate on the personal and social rather than the curriculum needs of the pupil. The unit's 'informal education' approach, although valuable for the young people, served to marginalize them from mainstream education, and removed schools' obligation to work with all young people. The schools' responsibility has been further eroded by extending provision for year 10 and 11 pupils to have a reduced National Curriculum, an increase in work placements and the right to attend further education college (School Standards and Framework Bill 1997).

The ability of government policy to influence school exclusions was apparent in New Zealand through a phenomenon known as 'Kiwi exclusions'. The 1989 New Zealand Education Act (Sect. 13/17) gave individual schools the legal responsibility of finding provision for excluded young people and providing guidance and counselling. Schools tried to avoid this by stating that the young person was 'a care and protection concern' and was therefore the responsibility of the Department of Social Welfare, who often refused to accept their definition. This resulted in a rise in referrals to the Department from 218 (1994/5) to 306 (1995/6). This situation was further compounded by the removal of geographically linked places and the introduction of a Privacy Act (1993) which restricted the flow of information between schools. This increased choice for some (in common with the aims of the English White Paper *Choice and Diversity (UK)* 1992), but in effect resulted in the 'loss' of thousands of young people from education (Gordon 1994). For example, in South Auckland 970 pupils were lost from school rolls in 1996 (Carruthers 1996).

A major area of legitimized exclusion from education in England is through the system of special educational needs (SEN). Despite government legislation (1976 and 1981 Education Acts, Green Paper 1997) recommending the integration of disabled young people into mainstream schools, this has been tempered by the proviso that integration should be dependent on the efficient use of resources. As a result, many schools and local authorities have used the possible additional expense of making schools accessible as an excuse for continuing segregation. Further, the system of SEN statementing, which enables disabled pupils to obtain additional resourcing and 'suitable' education, is a long professionalized process which further stigmatizes them and removes certain individual rights, such as freedom of choice and representation. The increased pressure on schools, particularly post-1988 (ERA), has been responsible for the disproportionate numbers of SEN-statemented young people being excluded (seven times the level of those without statements, DoE 1996) and the rapid rise in the number of referrals to 'special schools' of young people with 'emotional and behavioural difficulties'.

Some formal educational systems have, however, taken *inclusion* as a starting point for educational policy. The Gauteng Education Department's policy on special educational needs reflects the Salamanca Statement (Gauteng 1996) and the South African Bill of Rights (1995) by stating that 'inclusive education' aims 'to prepare all students for productive lives, as full, participating members of their communities'. It does this by ensuring that SEN pupils should be 'an integral part of the school community, therefore the responsibility should be on the school to create conducive learning environments' – what they call 'education for all together' (Gauteng 1996: 2). This approach uses a definition of SEN to encompass 'learners who are poor, who come from different cultural backgrounds, who are politically disadvantaged and who speak a different language from that of the school' (Gauteng 1996: 2).

Other policy has increased covert exclusion. Section 28 of the Local Government Act 1988 proposed a ban on 'the promotion of homosexuality' by local authorities with specific reference to schools, including the teaching in any mainstream school of the acceptability of homosexuality as a 'pretend' family relationship. Although the Act has never been activated, it has resulted in censorship and discrimination, and has enabled homophobic or unconfident professionals to ignore or – worse – negatively stereotype the home situations or sexualities of a significant proportion of the school population. It has also resulted in failure to challenge homophobic behaviour, resulting in 80 per cent of the 1,000 schools surveyed by Stonewall reporting homophobic bullying (Douglas *et al.* 1997).

Practice

The content and delivery of the National Curriculum and the increased bureaucracy and pressures of the test-driven education market-place have further exacerbated the problematic experience of formal education for many young people. Pupils may not be aware of the changes in policy which have affected their experience of school, but their comments show that teacher relations, curriculum content and reduced choice, such as lack of out-of-school activities, all rate highly in their reasons for 'dissatisfaction'.

Pupils' alienation from education is expressed in a number of ways, one of which is through self-exclusion, i.e. truancy. Overall, 10 per cent or 800,000 of the school population truant (UNISON/NASWE 1998). O'Keeffe's draft report for the DoE ('Truancy in English Secondary Schools', 1994) surveyed year 10 and 11 pupils in 150 schools in 20 local education authorities. The results showed that 'the incidence of truancy is shown to be greater than was believed by schools and motivated to a considerable extent by factors within the control of schools' (Miller, cited in O'Keeffe and Stoll 1995: 3). This view is supported by the findings of a nation-wide survey into truancy in Aotearoa, New Zealand, which recommends that 'schools recognize that some of the causes of truancy and poor behaviour may reside within the structures, organization, climate and programmes of school' (Education and Science Committee, New Zealand, 1995: 23, section 6.2.).

Teachers are experiencing increased alienation from the educational process. Bell (1995) discusses the 'deskilling' effect of recent legislation on teachers, who now have restricted opportunities, not only for creative and needs-led curriculum, but also to spend time building relationships with young people or to be involved in non-core curriculum subjects. The teacher's role is more clearly defined as the medium for the government-determined National Curriculum, and for the successful completion of pupils' attainment targets. A good relationship with teachers is an important determinant of pupils' sense of inclusion, and hence their levels of motivation and behaviour (Sanders and Hendry 1997; Rutter *et al.* 1979). The importance of a good relationship with teachers was evident in the comments of young people from a south Manchester exclusion project, who saw poor relations with teachers as being central to their reasons for alienation and often final exclusion from school. The young people wanted teachers to 'treat us equally' and 'treat us like they would treat themselves'. A sense of injustice also featured in the young people's comments: for example, not being 'allowed to speak', being blamed for something they did not do, and being excluded from decision-making. Several had been excluded as a result of violent behaviour directed at staff who they felt had treated them unfairly (Packham 1997). The O'Keeffe survey showed that 29 per cent of young people interviewed gave avoidance of an unpleasant teacher as a reason for truancy. The report *Exclusion from Secondary Schools* further supports O'Keeffe's findings by showing that 'good provision and especially good teaching are less likely to provoke indiscipline' (Ofsted 1996: 6), the cause of the majority of enforced exclusions.

The O'Keeffe study also showed that 'blanket' and post-registration truancy rose sharply in year 11, particularly among boys, and that most schools have a problem holding pupils of both sexes. The study's pupil questionnaires revealed that truancy was greatest in relation to particular subjects which were disliked by pupils (e.g. thought 'irrelevant' 36 per cent, 'unappealing' 22 per cent). An interest in the curriculum and its apparent relevance to the young people's present and perceived future opportunities also informs their sense of connection with formal education (Pearce and Hillman 1998). Radnor (1994) argues that for many young people the National Curriculum's emphasis on the theoretical (i.e. the ten compulsory National Curriculum subjects making up 70–80 per cent of the curriculum) limits the essential requirement for what Dewey calls the experiential learning of 'conceiving the connection between ourselves and the world in which we live' (Dewey 1966: 344).

It has been documented that schools with low levels of exclusion have a holistic approach, promoting a school ethos which values education (Commission for Racial Equality 1997; Ofsted 1996), and providing an education which is relevant to the needs and interests of its pupils: 'schools which exclude few pupils tend to be better ... at managing behaviour ... providing pastoral support and tailoring their curriculum to meet individual need' (Ofsted 1996: 6). There is, then, growing evidence that an inclusive curriculum reduces exclusion (Osler 1997). A review of what kind of curriculum is valuable to young people is therefore required, particularly identifying and improving areas of the curriculum affected by truancy and how it should be delivered.

Personal

Truancy and alienation from school is quite often seen merely as a symptom of disordered behaviour. Psychological explanations of behaviour have tended to view the school as unproblematic and 'anyone who recoiled from it as ipso facto deficient, or deviant' (O'Keeffe and Stoll 1995: 10) and therefore problematic and inadequate. Others argue that truants are in some ways deficient (Coldman 1995). Although it is likely that there will be individual factors relating to 'excluded' pupils, these may be as a result of alienation from education, which may have made them 'afraid, bored or confused' (Holt 1964: 1). Holt argues that the *process* of schooling is dehumanizing and alienating and is failing pupils. He advocates that schools should recognize and 'flunk unsuccessful methods, not the children' (Holt 1964: 8).

To concentrate solely on the personal as the main factor in exclusion is therefore to ignore the impact of the societal and institutional factors that affect school pupils. Research such as the O'Keeffe study has shown that individual factors alone do not explain levels of exclusion. The study showed that 'institutional factors are more significant than pupils' home background' (O'Keeffe 1994: 5), and that 'illness, bullying and home problems' were hardly mentioned by the pupils as a reason for truanting. Personal factors identified relate to the school's ability to deal with difference (e.g. racism) and teachers' attitudes towards personal circumstances. The young people interviewed from the school exclusion project had a sense of class difference from many teachers. They stated they were 'put down' if they were poor (e.g. couldn't buy books), were from single-parent families or did not do well at subjects, and consequently did not get into 'the teacher's good books' (Packham 1997).

It is also problematic to focus policy or practice on the most visible group of persistent truants, who may not be able to 'cope with the demands of schooling' (Coldman 1995: 77). This concentration on a small minority of pupils masks the true extent of truancy, another 80 per cent (Coldman 1995), and the reasons for non-attendance. Coldman argues against labelling truanting young people as having individual psychological, emotional and behavioural problems; rather, he argues that most young people who truant are not disaffected from school. Most pupils, whether truants or not, generally find school enjoyable and useful. This analysis sees truancy as a form of rational subject/school rejection, and therefore an indicator of curriculum effectiveness (Coldman 1995: 77).

Other theories have tried to place explanations for alienation within the home environment, although O'Keeffe's study found no connection between truancy and socio-economic status. Theories of cultural deprivation have also aimed to explain educational under-achievement, particularly of black and working-class young people, as the family's failure to socialize young people into the expected norms, language and culture of schools. In addition, the failure of black young people has been explained by theories of language deficit (Bernstein 1975), cognitive deficit (Eysenck 1970) and 'cultural capital' models (Bourdieu and Passeron 1977). These approaches have been rejected by Yekwai (1988), who locates the failure of black young people in schools as being a reflection of the derogatory values shown by society towards 'Afrikan' people. The finding of the OFSTED report (1996) also found that psychological factors or poor literacy were not the cause of the over-representation of African-Caribbean young people among exclusions, 'nor was it so obviously associated with deep-seated trauma as with many of the white children' (Ofsted 1996: 11). However, rather than identify possible explanations of exclusions within schools, the Ofsted report highlights the much higher percentage of black young people living with a lone parent than was the case with other groups. This is an example of the cultural deficit approach deflecting causal explanations of exclusion to factors external to the educational system and process. Sociological explanations for exclusion therefore challenge individual pathologizing and look for causal factors within schools themselves and within society.

Individual mechanisms for coping with alienation

In addition to outright avoidance of education, young people find means to show their disapproval or disconnectedness with disliked areas of schooling. The need for young people to establish individual and group identities in increasingly large and impersonal institutions has often been coupled with a lack of participation and involvement in the decisions that affect their lives. Responses to alienation range from passivity to physical withdrawal to 'active' disaffection (Pickles 1992). Gilmore identifies expressions of 'attitude', which can be apparent in what he calls 'stylized sulking' used by young people as 'messages of individual or collective autonomy in the face of authority' (Gilmore 1985: 113). He argues that this behaviour can become an educational block, as it is often perceived by teachers as 'skill deficiency' and used to label further and exclude the pupil.

Pupils' attitudes to school can therefore be seen to vary, depending on whether they see the whole or parts of their education as being of relevance. The DoE report (1996) showed that school itself had an important role in the lives of young people: most liked school and for many it had an important social function. Young people's approaches to school could therefore be determined by whether they are pro- or anti-school and pro- or anti-learning. Sue Lees (1993) proposes that girls who are pro-school and learning are academic and career-oriented and have high rates of success, particularly in single-sex schools (termed 'Boffin' girls by Blackman 1992). Those who were pro-school and anti-learning valued school mainly for its social aspects. She also identified three strategies which girls adopted to deal with 'abusive situations': *conformity* and resignation to the status quo, involving blaming themselves for uncomfortable situations; *avoidance*, where the young woman changes her behaviour or ignores the abusive behaviour, and *resistance*, which includes subversive activity, either verbal or collective (e.g. *The Little Red School Book* first produced 1969 [Hansen and Jensen 1969]) . Although Lees developed this framework in relation to girls, it is useful to consider in relation to behaviour in school by all young people. Particularly in co-educational schools, the suppression and exclusion of young women's experience is covert, and is imbedded in the 'hidden curriculum' (Sharpe 1976; Salisbury and Jackson 1996). This, coupled with lower self-confidence and socialized passivity still results in fewer young women becoming overtly resistant and disruptive. Young women's adoption of avoidance rather than confrontational behaviours may therefore explain the equal numbers of young males and women who truant – 36 per cent of girls abscond occasionally and 33 per cent of boys (Pearce and Hillman 1998) – but the low numbers of young women – 17 per cent – who are excluded (DoE 1996).

Public/societal factors

Sociological factors offer alternative explanations for exclusion and alienation which are not solely located within school, or with individual pupils, particularly in relation to the over-representation of particular groups. Such sociological explanations include pressure to conform to an 'anti-education' norm, economic factors and the apparent irrelevance of school to future prospects. One of the main functions of school has been to prepare for the world of work. School has not been able to keep up with the rapidly changing work environment, particularly to replace training for traditional manual and semi-skilled occupations for many working-class males (e.g. with new technology) or to cope with the demoralizing effects of high working-class unemployment (Chisholm 1990). This may be reflected in the fact that 83 per cent of excluded young people are male (DoE 1996). The relevance of school to present and future life is therefore an important factor in young people's attitudes to school.

If alienation from the school environment and curriculum as evident in self-exclusion and disruptive behaviour are the main causes of exclusion, it would be expected that similar groups of young people would be seen in both categories of exclusion (i.e. truants and excluded). This is the case for older white young people, but there are anomalies which require further investigation. For example, African-Caribbean pupils are six times more likely to be excluded but are not more likely to be persistent truants. Neither do they explain why girls truant equally to boys but few are excluded, or why disabled young people continue to be segregated in 'special schools' and are six times more likely to be excluded (DoE 1996). To explain such phenomena it is necessary to explore issues of societal discrimination and stereotyping that result in differing treatment and expectations (Green 1985) which permeate schools. These factors, forming part of the hidden curriculum, are hard to prove, and in fact were rejected as causes of truancy by O'Keeffe and Stoll (1995). However, they were very real factors for the excluded young people interviewed, who discussed the way they had been labelled at school. They wanted teachers to 'talk to you like a normal person, not a reject'.

The 'exclusion' of young women is an example of apparent success masking discrimination and hidden exclusion. Girls are now outperforming boys in all subjects except science (Abbott and Wallace 1997), resulting in the diversion of resources and attention to underachieving boys (see Secondary Heads Association 1997). These factors have masked continued subject specialism previously referred to as preferable for girls by the Crowther (1959) and Newsom (1963) Committees, and sex–role divisions which have been challenged but seemingly little changed since Mary Wollstonecraft's *A Vindication of the Rights of Women* (1792). This is particularly the case in relation to the educational experience of working-class girls and in relation to career aspirations and opportunities (Darling and Glendenning 1996).

Anomalies are also apparent in relation to African-Caribbean males whose case studies were found to be 'markedly different from those of others ... most of them were of average or above-average ability, but had been assessed by the schools as under-achieving' (Ofsted 1996: 11); they also have a higher 'staying-on' rate in post-16 education than white young people (CMEB 1998). These factors indicate that African-Caribbean young people have a desire to engage with education, but that there is a mismatch between their expectations and those of the teachers/schools.

The Swann Report pointed out that the situation of gypsy and traveller children 'illustrates to an extreme degree the experience of prejudice and alienation which faces other ethnic minority children' (Swann 1985: 6). This has resulted in many schools' refusal to accept traveller children. Of the 100,000 gypsies and travellers (Naylor *et al.* 1993), one fifth of primary school children and one third of secondary school-aged children have attendance figures below 50 per cent (Ofsted 1996); many others have not even been registered at school. Educators of travellers are concerned that the National Curriculum has narrowed the curriculum and concentrated on achieving high test scores at the expense of meeting diverse (cultural) needs.

Schools are a microcosm of society: they reflect dominant attitudes and values which are all too often based on stereotypes and assumptions of 'normality'. These values can result in practices which stigmatize rather than value difference, and exclude young people who are 'different' or who do not accept the content and practices of formal education. A reduction in exclusion therefore necessitates the provision of inclusive curriculum and methodology, not the problematizing of individual pupils.

Youth workers as critical practitioners with schools

Youth workers are increasingly involved with schools. In a time of reducing statutory youth services, schools have provided resources and direct access to youth workers' main client group. This shift has coincided with a growing awareness that youth work methods and relationships can be used effectively by schools and with 'disaffected' pupils in a range of settings. The school/youth work relationship, although potentially beneficial to all concerned, is, however, loaded with contradictions, particularly for the youth worker whose emphasis on the structural causes of exclusion may conflict with the schools' individual and family focus.

Nevertheless, youth workers, like school teachers, are 'first and foremost ... educators' (Rosseter 1987: 52). We share similar aims 'to facilitate and support young people's growth through dependence to interdependence by encouraging their personal and social education and helping them to take a positive role in the development of their communities and society' (National Youth Agency 1997: 25), and 'to provide a broad and balanced curriculum which promotes the spiritual, moral, cultural mental and physical development of pupils at school and of society and prepares pupils for the opportunities responsibilities and experiences of adult life' (ERA 1988).

Both teachers and youth workers are working to enable young people to reach their potential. What has increasingly separated us is that, while youth workers as informal educators use methodologies that apply the principles of empowerment, participation and anti-discriminatory practice (National Youth Agency 1990), teachers have become increasingly limited by policy and practice constraints. One of the dilemmas for youth work within formal settings is that we too might become similarly constrained.

The differing explanations for 'disaffection' pose particular contradictions for youth work with schools. The 'Pupils with Problems' Circulars (8–13, DoE 1994) recognized the role of the youth service in 'dealing with difficult pupils', and yet many youth workers have felt uncomfortable with their new role. This is particularly difficult when they recognize that *policy* may have resulted in the growing numbers of young people outside 'mainstream' education. The Circulars clearly see the young person, not the school, as the problem, and the role of the youth worker is to help the school control these young people, enabling them to stay on school roll. By working within schools where 'social control models have always prevailed', we are voluntarily succumbing to the 'control culture' that youth workers have fought hard to avoid (Jeffs and Smith 1994: 20). Further, youth work requires that pupils should identify their own needs, and negotiate the curriculum. This so-called 'child-centred' approach has been thought to 'encourage truancy' (DoE 1996: 19), and is contradictory to the centrally determined National Curriculum for schools. To work with excluded young people may necessitate adherence to this imposed and often irrelevant curriculum if the young person is to be reintegrated into school, when what is required is to consider the relevance and attractiveness of education .

A principle of youth work is to challenge inequality. However, to work with schools is to operate within an institutional framework which has perpetuated rather than challenged inequality (Bowles and Gintis 1976). For example, youth workers will be confronted with the differences between the medical model of disability (determining and perpetuating special educational needs) and the social approach of youth work, which recognizes structural causes of exclusion.

Youth work *practice* uses the same methods as those which have been labelled 'progressive education' and which have been blamed for increased levels of poor behaviour and truancy in schools (DoE 1996). This has been disputed by researchers who have shown that inclusive curriculum and participatory methodology reduces 'exclusion' (Osler 1997). Participatory youth work is characterized by individual or small group work, collaboration, discussion (critical dialogue) and negotiation. It recognizes the potential for young people to learn from experience and to make informed choices. 'It encourages young people to be critical in their responses to their own experience and the world around them' (National Youth Agency 1997: 25). The youth work focus on empowerment through participation is therefore compromised, as there is limited opportunity for power-sharing within schools, e.g. the negotiation of curriculum content, or involvement in decision-making. The youth work emphasis on criticism and change can also be viewed as confrontational to some formal educators.

Youth work uses the 'social model', based on individual rights and rejecting the problematizing of individuals without looking at the structural causes of their situation. *Personal* factors cannot therefore be isolated from *public* or societal ones. For many youth workers their role is one of liaison between the home/community and school, and as advocates for young people's rights. This may bring them into conflict with formal educators, who may see the needs of the many being disrupted by the behaviour of the few. Additionally, youth work with young people who reject and are consequently marginalized by school is at risk of being labelled a marginal service and not seen as an equal partner in the educational process.

Strategies

Youth workers have had to resolve the contradictions inherent in working as informal educators with school. They are clearer about their role and the important part they can play. Social and political education are increasingly being recognized as essential requirements for effective participation in society (Crick 1998), enabling youth workers as social and political educators to have recognized rather than marginalized roles within school. Curriculum changes may enable many teachers who have traditionally undertaken pastoral and informal education roles to have recognized curriculum time. These formal educators see education as what Bigelow calls a 'subversive activity', which should encourage critical thinking and so lead to social justice. He wants to be 'an agent of transformation, with my classroom as a centre of equality and democracy, an ongoing if small critique of the repressive social relations of the larger society' (quoted in Shannon 1992: 80). Freire (1972) calls this emancipatory education. These formal educators can be valuable youth work allies. The Social Exclusion Unit's report (1998) into school exclusion recognizes the value of such 'interagency' work between teachers and youth workers and calls for a 'joined-up' response to a 'joined-up' problem, identifying the multiplicity of causal factors both internal and external to the educational environment. The report's proposals, however, do not recommend holistic and structural strategies – rather, it suggests more publication of performance targets (in relation to exclusion), and seemingly punitive contracts (home–school agreements) backed up by legal punishment of offending parents (up to £1,000 fine). Its measures enable problematic and non-academic young people to be removed from mainstream education by the temporary suspension of the National Curriculum and an increased use of work experience placements. Neither of these measures looks at the structural causes of alienation discussed in this chapter. These measures will enable the young person to stay on the school roll (allowing the school to retain the pupil funding and have reduced exclusion figures) but will further exclude the young person within the school by stigmatizing them both as non-academic failures and as 'different'. This will continue to be the case while the success of schools is based on performance tables.

Conclusion

There is an interaction between the blades of the propeller of exclusion (see Figure 9.1), with some 'blades' being more prevalent at different times and for different groups. The report of the Social Exclusion Unit recognizes the complexity of factors affecting exclusions. This interrelation is supported by Sanders and Hendry (1997) who suggest that school ethos, pupil social backgrounds and low self-esteem interrelate strongly to create the dynamics of disruptive behaviour, the most common reason for exclusion. Although it is evident that external factors do influence young people's levels of success in school, there is no relationship between the socio-economic status of the school catchment area and the incidence of exclusion (Sanders and Henry 1997); rather, levels of exclusion seem to relate to the differing practices of local authorities (Children's Society 1998).

While male exclusion is a cause for concern and short-term strategies have been speedily introduced to tackle this overt issue, young women, disabled, lesbian and gay, working-class and black young people will continue to be the hidden excluded. These individuals may not be visible, as they may have adopted non-confrontational strategies of resistance which do not lead to legal exclusion. Some may be systematically segregated (disabled young people), and myriad young people's cultural and sexual experiences are excluded by the predominance of an imposed 'monoculture' (Gordon 1994). Some of these young people may be deemed by the excluding institutions to have 'succeeded' academically but at the expense of their personal identity and fulfilled potential.

Concern regarding increased and continuing exclusion necessitates the development of strategies based on acknowledging explanations of structural inequality both within and outside school. For youth workers, as critical practitioners, the ultimate dilemma is whether we are prepared to work within educational structures which perpetuate the discrimination we seek to challenge.

References

Abbott, P. and Wallace, C. (1997) *An Introduction to Sociology: Feminist Perspectives*, London: Routledge.

Audit Commission (1996), *Misspent Youth*, London: HMSO.

Bell, J. (1995) *Teachers Talking About Teaching*, Buckingham: Open University Press.

Bernstein, B. (1975) 'On the Classification and Framing of Knowledge', in *Class Codes and Control* vol. 3, London: Routledge and Kegan Paul, 85–115.

Bilton, T. (ed.) (1994) *Introduction to Sociology*, London: Macmillan.

Blackman, S. J. (1992) 'Pro-school pupils', *Youth and Policy* 38, 1–9.

Bourdieu, P. and Passeron, T. C. (1977) *Society and Culture*, London: Sage.

Bowles, S. and Gintis, H. (1976) *Schooling in Capitalist America*, London: Routledge and Kegan Paul.

Carruthers, Judge D.J. (1996) *Memorandum: South Auckland Youth Court*, New Zealand: Principal Youth Court Judge's Chambers.

Children's Society (1998) *No Lessons Learnt*, London: Children's Society.

Chisholm, L. (1990) *Childhood, Youth and Social Change,* London: Falmer Press.

Coldman, C. (1995) 'Rethinking the image of the truant', in D. O'Keeffe and P. Stoll (eds), *Issues in School Attendance and Truancy*, London: HMSO, 65–77.

Commission for Racial Equality (1997) *Exclusion from Secondary Schools and Racial Equality, A Good Practice Guide*, London: CRE and Prince's Trust.

Commission on the Future of Multi-Ethnic Britain (CMEB) (1998), *Consultative Document*, London: CMEB.

Crick, B. (1998) *Report of Advisory Group on Education for Citizenship and the Teaching of Democracy in Schools*, London: Qualification and Curriculum Authority.

Crowther Committee (1959) *15–18; A Report to the Central Advisory Council for Education (England)*, London: Ministry of Education.

Darling, J. and Glendinning, A. (1996) *Gender Matters in Schools*, London: Cassell.

Department of Education (1994) *Pupils with Problems*, Circulars 8–13/94, London: Publication Centre.

——(1996) *Permanent Exclusions from Schools in England (1995–6)*, London: Publication Centre.

Department of Education and Science (1988) *Education Reform Act*, London.

Dewey, J. (1915) *The School and Society*, Chicago: Chicago University Press.

Douglas, N., Warrick, I., Kemp, S. and Whitly, J. (1997) *Playing It Safe*, Health and Education Research Unit, Institute of Education, University of London.

Education and Science Committee (1995) *Inquiry into Children in Education at Risk through Truancy and Behavioural Problems*, Wellington, NZ: Ministry of Education.

Eysenck, H.J. (1970) *Intelligence and Education*, London: Temple Smith.

Freire, P. (1972) *Pedagogy of the Oppressed*, London: Penguin Books.

Gauteng (1996) *Discussion Document: Inclusion*, Department of Education, Gauteng, South Africa: Department of Education.

Gilmore, P. (1985) ' "Gimme room": school resistance, attitude and access to literacy', *Journal of Education*, 167, 111–28.

Gordon, C. (1994) *School Choice, Whose Choice?*, New Zealand: University of Canterbury.

Green, T. (1985) *Multi-Ethnic Teaching and Pupils' Self Concepts*, Annexe B in M. Swann, *Education for All. The Report of the Committee of Enquiry into the Education of Children from Ethnic Minority Groups*, London: HMSO.

Hansen, S. and Jensen, J. (1969) *The Little Red School Book*, London: Stage 1.

Hart, D. (1998) *Guardian*, 28 August, 4.

Holt, J. (1964) *How Children Fail*, Harmondsworth: Penguin.

Jeffs, T. and Smith, M. (1994) 'Young people, youth work and a new authoritarianism', *Youth and Policy*, 46 (autumn), 17–32.

Kilpatrick, R. and Barr, G. (1997) 'Suspension and Expulsion of Ulster Pupils', unpublished report for the DfEE, Belfast: School of Education, Queens University.

Lees, S. (1993) *Sugar and Spice*, Harmondsworth: Penguin.

Miller, P. (1995) 'Review of *Truancy in English Secondary Schools*', in D. O'Keeffe and P. Stoll (eds), *Issues in School Attendance and Truancy*, London: Pitman, 3–7.

Murray, C. (1990) *The Emerging British Underclass*, London: Institute of Economic Affairs.

National Youth Agency (1990) *Ministerial Statement of Purpose*, from the Second Ministerial Conference, London: NYA.

——(1997) *Mapping the Youth Work Sector*, London: NYA.

Naylor, S., Waterson, M. and Whiffin, M. (1993) *The Education of Gypsy and Traveller Children: Action Research and Co-ordination*, Hatfield: University of Hertfordshire Press.

Newsom Committee (1963) *Half Our Future. A Report to the Central Advisory Council for Education (England)*, London: Ministry of Education, 52–65.

OFSTED (1996) *Exclusion from Secondary Schools 1995/6*, London: The Stationery Office.

——(1998) *The Education of Travelling Children*, London: The Stationery Office.

O'Keeffe, D.J. (1994) *Truancy in English Secondary Schools*, London: HMSO.

O'Keeffe, D. and Stoll, P. (1995) *Issues in School Attendance and Truancy*, London: Pitman.

Osler, A. (1997) *Exclusion from School and Racial Equality*, London: Commission for Racial Equality.

Packham, C. (1997) 'Informal Education with Schools', unpublished report, Manchester Metropolitan University: Department of Applied Community Studies.

Pearce, N. and Hillman, J. (1998) *Wasted Youth: Raising Achievement and Tackling Social Exclusion*, London: Institute of Public Policy Research.

Pickles, T. (1992) *Dealing with Disaffection*, Harrow: Longman.

Radnor, H. (1994) *Across the Curriculum*, London: Cassell.

Rosseter, B. (1987) 'Youth Workers as Educators', in T. Jeffs and M. Smith (eds), *Youth Work*, Basingstoke: Macmillan Education.

Rutter, M. (1979) *Fifteen Thousand Hours. Secondary Schools and Their Effects on Children*, Somerset: Open Books Publishing.

Salisbury, J. and Jackson, D. (1996) *Challenging Macho Values*, London: Falmer Press.

Sanders, D. and Hendry, L. B. (1997) *New Perspectives in Disaffection*, London: Cassell.

Secondary Heads Association (1997) *Can Boys Do Better?*, London: SHA.

Shannon, P. (ed.) (1992) *Becoming Political. Readings and Writings in the Politics of Literacy Education*, Portsmouth: Heinemann Education.

Sharpe, S. (1976) *Just Like a Girl*, Harmondsworth: Penguin Books.

Social Exclusion Unit (1998) *Truancy and School Exclusion*, London: The Stationery Office.

Swann, M. (1985) *Education for All. The Report of the Committee of Enquiry into the Education of Children from Ethnic Minority Groups*, London: HMSO.

UNISON and National Association of Social Workers in Education (NASWE) (1998) *Joint Submission to the Social Exclusion Unit*, London: UNISON.

Wollstonecraft, M. (1975) [1792] *A Vindication of the Rights of Women*, Harmondsworth: Penguin.

Yekwai, D. (1988) *British Racism: Miseducation and the African Child*, London: Karnak House.

10 Sparring partners

Conflicts in the expression and treatment of self-harm

Helen Spandler and Janet Batsleer

Self-harm can be viewed as a contradictory and ambivalent activity. The concepts of ambivalence (to take a term from psychoanalysis) or contradiction (to take a term from dialectics) may be critical exploratory devices to look at the expression and treatment of self-harm. Self-harm foregrounds ambivalences and conflicts which are at the heart of our professional and theoretical struggles. Instead of these tensions being kept in mind and practice, they tend to turn into socially powerful dualisms. Rappaport (1981) uses dialectics in order to understand and recognize that we are pulled in two ways at once, and argues that we need to pursue paradoxes in practice. He argues that we need to pay attention to different and apparently opposed poles of thought. To pursue one apparently dominant theme or 'solution' can create unintended negative consequences by ignoring the other side. We can see this happening in treatment and responses to self-harm.

In this chapter, we are concerned with the identification and analysis of these conflicts, and look at the different arenas where these are played out. We will look at institutional and professional responses to self-harm, the self-harm/survivor movement and the discussions of self-harm in the music press. We are concerned with how much work seems to go into keeping these various domains and conflicts separate. We raise the question of where and how these various contradictions and ambivalences may be brought together and worked with.

Criticism and opposition have been an integral part of the psychiatric 'field' since its earliest developments. Crossley uses Bourdieu's term 'field' to emphasize the 'fluidity, dynamism, competition and conflicts which characterize the social space around psychiatry' (Crossley 1998: 877). We argue that in these different arenas particular conflicts and dualisms are highlighted, certain issues are spoken about and addressed or included, and others are excluded. Thus, for example, the survivor discourse articulates particular issues which have been difficult to express in professional/institutional settings, and popular culture may allow other conflicts to be expressed which are marginalized in other fields. Popular culture is an area that the mental health field would not ordinarily consider, as it is outside the psychiatric field of expertise. However, this arena is important in that it is (by definition) widely available.

The 1960s and 1970s saw popular critiques of 'schizophrenia' and 'asylums' (e.g. Laing 1967; Goffman 1968) and the beginnings of the emergence of the modern user movement in, for example, the Mental Patients' Union in the early 1970s. This was followed in the 1980s by critiques of traditional treatments of eating disorders which offered a political feminist critique read by a mass audience. The late 1980s and 1990s have seen the pathologization and psychiatrization of hearing voices being questioned by people who hear voices. In the 1990s there has been a proliferation of alternative accounts of self-harm and a critique of treatment, both by survivors and by their allies.

The mental health user movements – such as Survivors Speak Out and the Self-Harm Network in Britain – give public voice to experiences of distress and oppression which are more usually seen as private experiences. The user movements enable their members to speak as experts on their own lives, rather than remaining the 'objects' of the expert-knowledge claims of others. The discourses of survivors and users of the psychiatric system set up a counter-discourse to both psychology and psychiatry. They hold up a mirror to those powerful experts, inviting professionals to see themselves as involved in the construction of distress and despair, rather than outside it.

The movement of speaking out in relation to self-harm is building on earlier movements, and in particular oppositional practices in welfare and psychiatry. This participates in a recent trend in survivor organizations to 'self-manage' and 'control' their experiences which have been pathologized, rather than to seek 'expert' help or even necessarily to change. Thus, the Hearing Voices Network advises voice-hearers on how to 'cope with' and 'live with' their voices and even to integrate them into their lives. The Manic Depression Fellowship looks towards strategies of 'self-management' of moods – 'highs' and 'lows' – by people with manic depression (Manic Depression Fellowship 1997). In addition, various drug agencies (pushed by drug users themselves) have moved towards accepting that young people will take drugs and to developing models of harm reduction. Similarly, the gay movement is campaigning for the rights of gay men to control their sexual activities and critique state/medical intervention and regulation. Some information and literature from gay men has suggested that in order to tackle HIV/AIDS we need to recognize that gay men may still have unprotected sex with their partners, and that intervention must work with this rather than promote a narrow and 'pure' strategy of, for example, 'always using a condom' (Mitchell 1998). Similarly, the Self-Harm Network aims to support and inform self-harmers and their allies about (self) harm minimization, the provision of 'safety kits', looking after wounds, living with scars.

This could reflect a therapeutic and social pessimism and/or realism. Or alternatively, it could be seen as a response to the failure of psychiatric and therapeutic interventions by those on the receiving end. In challenging their status as the objects of the knowledge of professionals and scientists, the activists in these organizations call on and lay claim to people's individual and collective 'agency' and 'rights'. In doing so they are building on the political achievements not only of the movements against oppression in psychiatry, but also of other new social movements, particularly the gay movement and the women's liberation movements (Wilton, in Griffin 1995). Eating disorder groups and self-harmers draw most explicitly on feminist discourses around control and the body.

Mental health is about the most private troubles, not only interpersonal but intrapersonal. Common occurrences, such as cutting oneself, are also felt as deeply individual and usually very private activities. It is, for the person who self-harms, 'my own special creation' (Spandler 1996: 55). The separation of the political and the personal has to be challenged, if there is to be a politics of mental health at all, in the same way that feminist theorists and activists have challenged the separation of the public and private spheres as the legitimate basis for political activity. Other separations or dualisms – the inner and outer; self and other; mind and body; individual and social – also need to be challenged. Self-harm can be understood in terms of the struggle of power and resistance.

Power/resistance; control/risk

The organization of psychiatric services has historically excluded people who experience mental health problems from discussions about the meaning and understanding of their experiences. Self-harm is one recent example of a continuing debate and struggle over the definition, control and treatment of experience and behaviour.

If power not only restrains but produces, in this instance the control and management of self-harm has produced a number of new energizing and articulate accounts from self-harmers themselves. The misunder-standings and lack of adequate support to self-harmers and, in particular, punitive responses have inadvertently created a tension between professionals and self-harmers which has come to the fore in resistances to adverse treatment, with self-harmers coming together, gaining support from each other, producing and developing survivor-written information and campaigning materials (as exemplified by the National Self-Harm Network). It is the labelling, treatment and control of the phenomenon of 'self-harm' (its psychiatrization) that has made possible a 'movement' of people who self-harm and their allies to assert their right to exist – their identity, rights and dignity.

What professionals might see as a 'helping' intervention can be experienced as invasive, punishing, patronizing and controlling. At the worst end of this it can replicate feelings of powerlessness and abuse. It is the control aspect of self-harm which survivors' discourses empha-size. It is therefore important to recognize this in reactions and treatments to the behaviour. The Self-Harm Network published a sheet designed for self-harmers to use which is designed to support their treatment and to assist the management of their care by Accident and Emergency departments. It is addressed 'To the triage nurse' and contains a section: 'What you need to know to make my treatment as effective as possible'. The person carrying the sheet can tick boxes which contain statements such as: 'I need you to examine my injury in a private room'; 'I am happy for students to observe or treat me'; 'I would like to see a psychiatrist.' Each of the statements concerns the detail of interaction in the hospital, and identifies a moment in which control might be taken away from the person who self-harms and where medical power might be abused. If we understand this dynamic of control, it will come as no surprise that self-harm occurs frequently in controlling environments such as prisons, special hospitals, secure units and psychiatric wards.

There are powerful links to be found between activism in relation to violence against women and the work of the National Self-Harm Network. Both movements share a concern with emphasizing the strength and creativity of people who have experienced violence, and move from a discourse of 'victim' to a discourse of 'survivors'. It is the ambivalence between control and risk which is most directly addressed in the survivor literature, and in this emphasis it builds on the knowl-edges developed in the women's movement. Self-injury is seen as a practical way of coping in intense distress, potentially a way of averting suicide. The publications of the National Self-Harm Network are intensely practical in tone. They answer straightforward questions in a straightforward manner, with little room for ambiguity.

There is a significant strand in survivors' accounts about self-injury which makes a powerful connection with sexual abuse and other physical assaults. These are all situations where power has been exercised and freedom taken away. We need to understand the 'means of action available to agents in specific situations of action' (Hindess 1982: 506). People in subordinate positions have often been recognized as adept at converting whatever resources they possess into some degree of control over the conditions of their existence. .

Various forms of self-harm may be seen as a way for individuals to assert a sense of agency and resist disciplinary practices which position them, among other things, as 'young', 'patients', 'women', 'prisoner', 'abused' or 'personality-disordered'. Where the public and private, self and other seem to invade each other; where a person feels controlled by others, by situations, emotions or memories, here the act of self-harm may enable them to experience themselves as agentic, it may give them 'private space' and give them a sense of 'selfhood' and personal autonomy. This is exemplified in statements by self-harmers and people with eating disorders, who, in relation to the activity, say things like: 'it's mine', 'it's something for me'. Accounts from self-harmers and people with eating disorders have articulated various benefits of the behaviour, such as offering safety, certainty, security, protection and comfort. Self-harm, like eating disorders, provides individuals with a sense of power, control and achievement through the individualized and often secret expression of conflict.

In *Domination and the Arts of Resistance*, Scott (1990) gives an account of the 'hidden transcripts' of subordinates as compared to 'official transcripts'. Hidden transcripts take place 'offstage', beyond the direct observation of power-holders. The public transcript offers apparent consensus and deference, whereas the hidden version may be an articulation of dissatisfaction. The hidden transcript is usually, however (ideally), communicated with other subordinates in order to gain strength and an experience of opposition. Self-harm may itself represent an inability and impossibility of validating feelings and experiences with others to offer 'shared transcripts'. This sharing is what organizations such as the Self-Harm Network seek to achieve. Self-harm seems almost, by its very nature, to be isolated, atomized and individualized. It may be that for people who self-harm the act itself must be such as to give the person doing it a sense of opposition. It seems to be the action of, for example, cutting or eating (or not eating) which gives a sense of agency. The secrecy involved in self-harming and bulimia/bingeing may contribute to its sense of (individual) power. In addition, accounts from survivors of eating disorders and self-harm have often emphasized the sense of achievement/pride they get from the activity. Yet, paradoxically, the behaviour may appear 'out of control' to others.

Self/other; individual/social

Self-harm may be seen as an action taken in order to actively control overwhelming feelings, situations and memories ('cutting myself takes away the pain', 'it stops me remembering'). The self-harm plays out/re-enacts power/control dynamics. The individual harms themselves, thereby becoming (to themselves) both the abuser and the abused. The self-harm actually enacts the breakdown in self/other and joins in with the attack on the self. Interventions, treatments and institutional responses can reinforce the need for such strategies by taking control away from the individual. Conventional intervention both infantalizes the self-harmer and exacerbates the very feelings which are thought to contribute to the behaviour.

One particularly compelling account of self-harm is a psychody-namic interpretation in which the 'self' and the 'other' are seen as entangled in a destructive way. The attack on the 'self' is an attack on the hostile introjected 'other' (Collins 1996). Self-harm can be seen as a way of forcing a break, forcing a separation between the self and a hostile social network in a self-protective and, paradoxically, also potentially life-threatening way. Where interpersonal difficulties have become so 'cut off' from their social origins and the individual so cut off from any relational networks of understanding/empathy, an activity such as self-harm becomes an attempted 'solution' to conflict, whereby the individual literally cuts themselves up in order to survive.

Mind/body

'In the reality of practice, the body is never outside history, and history is never free of bodily presence and effects on the body' (Connell 1987: 87). The struggle for control and power has become increasingly sited in (and on) the individual body. Various inter-, intra- and transper-sonal tensions and conflicts are literally inscribed on the body. Tensions expressed about the self/other; inner/outer; public/private; individual/social; life/death meet in the body, and in the practice of self-harm. At the same time, it may be that self-harm involves an extreme separation of body from self: the self as a courageous spirit and subject, attacking the stubborn object and thing, the body. The body becomes like an object; the regressive site for relationship; a substitute for relationship; and even the sole means of relating. Parts of the body become a site for the projection of emotions and social conflict.

Life/death

Ambivalence is a turning in two directions simultaneously. It means holding at least two contradictory and opposing feelings towards the self, which is torn in two by the pressures of life. It can be argued that the same ambivalences are present in self-harm and attempted suicide, and that the action of self-harm moves us towards a life-affirming resolution whereas attempted suicide moves in the direction of death. The fighting partners in this ambivalence have a number and variety of names. They include: love/hate; control/risk; silence/speech; pain/comfort; excitement/numbing; life/death. There is nothing unusual about this ambivalence; it is a normal phenomenon, in the sense that the destruction of the self at the hands of conflicting and untameable impulses is a possibility available to all humans.

Traditional medical/psychiatric accounts attempt to separate self-harm and attempted suicide, but only on grounds of suicidal intention. The distinction appears to be between a 'real' suicide attempt and a pretend one. Self-harm has been traditionally viewed as a 'failed' suicide, a 'suicidal gesture' or, technically, a 'parasuicide'. This has been recently challenged by the self-harm/survivor movement, who emphasize the meanings inherent in self-harm itself.

Similarly, early theories about bulimia were minimal and mainly confined to seeing it as a 'failed' anorexia. What seems to matter in terms of intervention and response is distinctions and polarities, such as moral ones like the deserving/undeserving, and divisions between preconceptions of life and death. The degree of nearness to death is what enables categorization and the split between 'the serious attempt on one's own life' and, for example, a 'teenage prank'. Survivor organizations seem to focus on pressurizing for moving away from prevention towards a toleration and acceptance of 'risk'/danger, which challenges such split professional responses.

Self-harm survivor accounts also seem to make an unambiguous separation between self-harm and attempted suicide, but this time by emphasizing that: 'Self-harm is about survival, not suicide' (Pembroke (1994). Thus, they try to resolve the life/death ambivalence in favour of life.

Perhaps this distinction is too neat. For example, in a curious way suicide attempts which do not lead to death can also lead to survival, and not only after the event. Attempting suicide by overdosing, for example, is about taking a decisive step, a decisive action to resolve an unbearable ambivalence, an impassable block. In addition, self-harm may be caught up in many ways with suicidal thoughts, feelings and outcomes. We are not arguing that there is no distinction between self-harm and suicide, and in particular it is important to recognize self-harm as an act not necessarily linked with suicide. However, artificial distinctions blur both the emotional and social issues which underlie both attempted suicide and self-harm.

Self-harm and attempted suicide are profoundly ambivalent and contain both self-destructive and life-affirming meanings. This ambivalence has begun to be addressed in some discourses around self-harm. Survivors' discourses represent self-harm as both distress/self-damage and as a multi-purpose coping mechanism. Some psychodynamic interpretations have also expressed the importance of the contradiction, e.g. 'While self-harm may be about survival, it is also about failing to survive' (Collins 1996 : 469).

Institutionalized responses

Deserving/undeserving; care/punishment; approval/disapproval

Most welfare discourses have a strong regulatory aspect, usually concerned with prevention. The survivors' movement has challenged this in favour of an awareness of the meanings of self-harm and toleration of risk. Self-harm brings out dual and split responses in treatments and interventions. The formation of a caring response to self-harm may appear clear, but so is its sparring partner: punishment. The punishment side of this conflict has been highlighted by survivors. The punitive nature of in-patient admission for anorexia and eating disorders, 'teaching women a lesson', has been noted, and more recently the Self-Harm Network has campaigned against various punishing practices in the 'treatment' of self-harm such as. stitching wounds without anaesthetic, threats and insults.

According to Louise Pembroke, definitions of self-harm are reminiscent of the old distinction between the deserving and the undeserving. Some types of self-harm meet with widespread social approval, others with stigma:

Socially acceptable forms of self-harm include: excessive smoking, drinking, exercise, liposuction, bikini line waxing, high heels and body piercing. Western societies endorse and promote women's assaults on their bodies by dieting. This form of self-harm is encouraged by cultural and gender expectations and pressures. More women die in the United States as a result of eating distress than of AIDS ... The socially acceptable range of self-harm clearly does not include self-cutting, burning, smashing bones and pouring toxic substances over or into our bodies. This is normally referred to by the medical profession as self-mutilation, more commonly 'Deliberate Self-Harm'.

(Pembroke 1994: 2)

It could be claimed that self-harm involves a 'DIY' non-commodi-fied act rather than market purchases of 'beauty treatments' or 'retail therapy'. It has often been argued that eating disorders produce an exaggerated parody of women's culturally specified body size and a protest against being controlled. Self-harm seems to take this sense of distortion a step further. Eating disorders use culturally sanctioned concerns about food, weight, dieting and body shape. Self-harm increasingly uses the self against itself, by whatever means necessary.

Another related split Pembroke has identified here is that between approval and disapproval. The discourse of listening and caring also enacts themes around love/hate, and this ambivalence is split in profes-sional responses to self-harm, and in regulatory accounts of the 'clients' who are listened to and cared for: as cold recipients of warm contact, to be sure, but also as manipulative, attention-seeking bullies who deserve nothing but contempt.

In our last pattern, we look at those who could be said to give suicidal behaviour a really bad name. This is because they use it directly as emotional blackmail. In many ways what they do is very simple. They take tablets to get attention and to change the emotional attitudes of their lover, relatives, friends or whoever does not comply with their wishes. They manage their lives by manipulating other people.

(Eldrid 1988: 52)

Material written from experiences at a therapeutic community, the Henderson Hospital, looks at the how institutional responses provide relationships based on power and control, not empathy and under-standing:

Hierarchical and authoritarian arrangements are observable in all hospitals and ... may serve to increase the likelihood of the enactment of complementary relationships of victim or perpetrator based on a power differential between patients and their carers. As a result, the situation serves to maintain the status quo, since tension is discharged more readily interpersonally, between patient and staff or staff and staff, than it is contained intra psychically by the patient and staff.

(Norton and Dolan 1996: 80)

Many psychiatric hospitals/institutions may in effect mirror the individual self-harming,

in that they tend to display only a narrow repertoire of relatively inflexible responses, which serve the objectives of wider society. Unwittingly, certain of these institutional responses ... can serve to escalate rather than ameliorate such behaviour, to the detriment of both the patient and the institution.

(Norton and Dolan 1996: 77)

These responses, it is argued, merely serve to collude with one or other side of the patient's internal conflict, producing an interpersonal enactment between patient and staff and/or between staff and staff who take up extreme and opposing positions either 'for' or 'against' the patient.

Unfortunately, survivors' accounts are not immune from these difficulties. Self-harmers' accounts may also produce and reinforce various splits and divisions which may continue to mirror and amplify already existing powerful dynamics. This discourse often positions self-harmers as the only ones who 'really' understand self-harm (although they may readily admit that 'if I knew why I do it, I wouldn't need to do it'). Thus, they position 'others' (e.g. professionals, family) as non self-harmers and as therefore 'not understanding'. This can be viewed as reinforcing an 'us and them' division and may actually serve to cut off any support and solidarity.

Speech/silence

The Samaritans find that callers often say after an initial encounter that they feel much better for talking. Although their problems are still far from solved, the callers no longer feel so alone in their despair and anxiety. When you are out in the cold, feeling suicidal and seeking help, the warm response of another human being could save you from freezing to death.

(Eldrid 1988: 146)

The ambivalence between silence and speech is clearly resolved in favour of speech. The need for a warm response when you are freezing is undeniable. However, all too often professional talk about listening silences the content of the conversation, turning it into a mute cry of need. So loud is the voice of the professional's concern that s/he interrupts and seeks to present an alternative agenda. The invitation 'speak or confess' may serve the professional's need to know and may leave the self-harmer unprotected and vulnerable.

Survivor discourses, as well as emphasizing the need to reassert control, also recognize the need to break silence and to speak about the unspeakable, rather than simply to write it on the body.

Self-harm is as taboo as sexual abuse has been. For those who live with it, there is much fear and shame in talking about it. For those who work with self-harm, there is great reluctance to face it beyond the stereotype ... Self-harm is a sane response when people are gagged in order to maintain the social order. Self-harm mirrors what we don't want to acknowledge. Explosive feelings implode. Our emotional corset cannot hold the pain any longer so it bursts. Self-harm is about self-worth, self-preservation, lack of choices and coping with the unacceptable.

(Pembroke 1994: 1)

Pembroke identifies the unacceptability of many of the conditions individuals have no choice but to cope with. It is both the unacceptability and the lack of choice that contribute to self-harm as a response. What might happen if those explosive feelings, imploding in self-harm, were turned outwards and were able to be spoken in the face of the unacceptable? Eating disorders and self-harm have also been described as a covert way to express unacceptable emotions such as, in particular, anger. Thus, in some ways they operate as a means by which an individual does not communicate their dissatisfaction, frustration and anger. It is often said that eating disorders and self-harm are used when a person lacks the means to communicate in words. The ambivalence between silence and speech, public and private, is extremely hard to resolve. Self-harm is, on the whole, an unspoken action, a secret. There is a fear of communicating distress, perhaps because it increases vulnerability. When people who self-harm get together, it can be witnessed that the articulation of feelings and hearing others speak seems to equate with having the defence of silence and the privacy/specialness of the self-harm removed. This therefore operates as a tension within and between self-harmers as well as between a self-harmer and their helper, who will 'want to know what's wrong'.

Popular culture: the expression of despair/elation

There exists a long cultural tradition which celebrates the release, relief, comfort and ecstasy of dying. Death has been seen as the final 'limit' to be transgressed:

> Now more than ever seems it rich to die,
> To cease upon the midnight with no pain,
> While thou art pouring forth thy soul abroad
> In such an ecstasy!
>
> (John Keats, 'Ode to a Nightingale')

> To die will be an awfully big adventure.
>
> (J.M. Barrie, *Peter Pan*)

Nor was this only a masculine tradition. Sylvia Plath's poetry celebrated domestic pain, cutting herself in the kitchen, with pleasure. In her poem *Cut* (1965) the excitement and thrill of cutting are vividly represented. The vegetable knife flashes and cuts the top of the skin instead of an onion. The poem describes the hinge of skin, dead white, and then the vivid red plush, conjuring all the attraction and fear associated with wanting to see the blood.

Joni Mitchell sang about the needle

> underneath the skin
> an empty space to fill in.

The blade and the needle have their attractions: they both threaten death and give access to 'that red plush'. Such cultural forms are not pathological (although Plath, being a woman, has sometimes been considered so): they are considered high art, and Peter Pan is one of the most popular heroes of children's fiction.

Most media coverage of self-harm has been unsurprisingly sensationalist and reminiscent of familiar moral panics. The public gaze has voyeuristically turned to self-harm – long available as a practice in the culture, after all: the latest piece of subjectivity with which to control, scrutinize, treat and now in turn 'give voice to'.

However, the discussion of issues of self-harm in the music press offers an indication that it is not only to professional/clinical spaces in the culture that we might look when we are in search of a social/political framework. Professional discourses are very much concerned with methods of helping, and each will offer its own technology of care, from the listening ear to methods of behaviour modification. The content of what is said to 'the listening ear' can too readily become marginalized. Paradoxically, it is through the nihilist assertions of Richey James, formerly of the Manic Street Preachers – 'I know I believe in nothing but it is my nothing' – that a discussion of the meaning of self-harm in the context of prevailing social relations briefly emerged. The rejection of prevailing values and the claim that the only truth and basis for living is to be found in an act of courageous self-definition in the face of meaninglessness has provoked a number of questions. What elements can form such courageous acts of 'self-definition'? How do these acts symbolize the prevailing social conditions of which they are a part? What forces of destruction are ranged against such acts?

If self-harm seemed to remain taboo for many people who worked professionally with it, the same has not been true elsewhere in culture. The music industry and the music press particularly were entering a two-year period in which discussions of suicide and self-harm were rarely absent from their coverage and their letters columns. In 1994 Kurt Cobain joined 'that stupid club' of Hendrix, Morrison, Moon and Vicious, and shot himself. Almost a year later Richey James disappeared. He had achieved notoriety after carving '4 REAL' into his arm during an interview in 1991 'to show that we are not just a gimmick'. In 1992, the Manic Street Preachers' American tour ended with a tribute to Allen Ginsberg, with a playing of Ginsberg's 'Howl', itself written on a psychiatric ward.

The discourses surrounding both the music of the Manic Street Preachers and the disappearance of Richey James provide a further countervailing discourse to that of professionals. They are also very distinct from the discourses of the survivors' movement, more philosophical and less practical. They provide a powerful instance of popular culture providing a framework of expression and a space for debate in ways that were potentially affirming for survivors and critical of the culture in which 'everything just seems for sale'. The music of the Manic Street Preachers is exhilarating rock which doesn't evade or give in to the pain the lyrics speak about.

The Manic Street Preachers were formed in 1986 at the height of the Thatcher years. They talked about their music in an intellectual/poetic tradition that drew on Mirabeau, Solanos, Ginsberg, William Burroughs and Nietzche. The despair and the pain are that of the outsider who stands apart from the everyday and judges it as bankrupt. The music moves outside the common themes of pop to themes that are not frequently found in rock music: the evils of corporate banking, Third World deforestation, eating disorders, the tobacco industry.

The most powerful song on the album *The Holy Bible* is an anorexic's elated celebration of her achievement in reaching 4st 7lb. It is here, in a way that is quite unusual, that the elation found in the despair/elation contradiction is spoken and addressed:

> I don't mind the horror that surrounds me
> Self worth scatters
> Self esteem's a bore
> I long since moved to a higher plateau
> This discipline's so rare so please applaud
> Just look at the fat scum who pamper me so
> yeh 4st 7, an epilogue of youth
> such beautiful dignity in self abuse
> (Manic Street Preachers, *The Holy Bible*)

In linking self-harm and cutting with anorexia, Richey James is challenging some of the firmly created gender boundaries which link suicide with masculinity and self-harm and eating disorders with femininity. Many contributions to the discussion that occurred in the music press suggest that there is no social or political basis for the distress expressed in this music and by young listeners There is certainly little conventional evidence of personal experience of social deprivation through, for example, unemployment and poverty. There could be a modern concern with previously unexpressed dissatisfactions with masculinity. It is arguable that the 'common-sense' assumption that men tend to commit suicide and women to harm themselves may have been reproduced in earlier cultural forms (as exemplified by Keats and Plath above). However, it is interesting that here it has been a young man who has powerfully represented feelings around self-harm. The engagement with gender, sexuality and self/identity is caught up with a sexual politics in a way that is very different from the masculine heroism associated with outsider status in beat culture. However, the heroic element is not lost altogether. It is possible to recognize an elitist triumphalist strand in some accounts of self-harm. After all, it requires a quite particular courage. The music and presence of Richey – his body emaciated and his chest slashed – speak something which is repressed elsewhere in discourses surrounding self-harm. In focusing on the pain, and making the pain visible, the exhilaration, the thrill, the elation involved in finding a physical limit, the pleasure of self-inflicted pain, become visible too.

Following Richey's disappearance, both the *New Musical Express* and *Melody Maker* were inundated with letters:

> The letters that have reached *NME* since Richey disappeared suggest that there is another huge constituency of fans out there – the cutters, anorexics and bulimics. In the past, there's been no one to represent these individuals in popular culture. Cutting and fasting had traditionally been a hidden thing, as the sufferers tried to exercise control over their lives or to express inner rage. Many of these people plainly felt they were sharing a secret with Richey. He made them feel better, less like freaks ... Now that he's gone their levels of anxiety, as revealed to this paper, are too awful to contemplate.
>
> (*New Musical Express*, April 1995)

In an attempt to contemplate the distress and respond to it, *Melody Maker* ran a special edition jointly with the Samaritans called 'From Despair to Where?' in which the issues of depression and despair were discussed. There is a striking contradiction throughout this discussion. On the one hand, Richey James is seen as speaking for and about young people's experience of a barbarous culture; on the other hand is the view that clinical depression must be recognized and treated as such, and not glamorized. From one point of view, the discussions of nihilism and philosophy are irrelevant at best and potentially dangerous at worst. There is a sort of momentary confluence when it is acknowledged that the flood of letters the paper received – mostly from girls – demands the recognition that depression is a common experience.

The distress associated with self-harm is made apparent in psycho-logical and social work responses to the issue. However, we can also view the other side of this as the repression of delight/elation/relief which, while accompanying the experience of self-harm, does not appear in these accounts. The popular culture we have discussed may enable the recognition of what is repressed in professional – and even many survivor – accounts (although Lefevre 1996 is an exception).

Summary

Self-harm involves important ambivalences, conflicts and paradoxes. Different, often competing, discourses allow particular conflicts and dualism to be addressed and often replicated. For example, professional discourses address and enact issues of power and control; management and prevention; reason and understanding, speech and talking, despair and disorder, etc. Survivor discourses address themes such as comfort, relief, control, survival, hope, risk. Popular culture may express exhilaration, thrill, pain, excitement and joy as well as panic and despair.

We are arguing here that we need to work with these various conflicts and ambivalences at all levels – personal, professional, institutional and political. In terms of bringing together the personal 'internal' conflicts, ambivalences and 'splits', psychoanalytic understanding may be deemed appropriate. However, this also needs to apply to institutions, professionals and social structures which exemplify and perpetuate particular conflicts and contradictions.

Where can all these polarities and divisions begin to be brought together and taken seriously? Where are the social, cultural and political spaces in which this could happen? Is there a politics which challenges the coercive and abusive patterns of relationship to which self-harm is a response, and which can speak about pain and elation, life and death, power and resistance, etc., a practice that can really get under our skins? To work with both sides of the conflicts expressed in the act and treatment of self-harm means developing practices which challenge too private an account of attempted suicide and self-harm, and enable an address to the social and political questions with which self-harm is implicated.

References

Barrie, J.M. (1992) [1911] *Peter Pan and Wendy, or, The Boy Who Would Not Grow Up*, London: Hodder and Stoughton Folio Society.

Collins, D. (1996) 'Attacks on the Body: How Can We Understand Self-Harm?', *Psychodynamic Counselling*, 2, 463–75.

Connell, R.W. (1987) *Gender and Power*, Cambridge: Polity Press.

Crossley, N. (1998) 'R.D. Laing and the British anti-psychiatry movement: a socio-historical analysis', *Social Science and Medicine*, 47(7), 877–89.

Eldrid, J. (1988) *Caring for the Suicidal*, London: Constable.

Goffman, E. (1968) *Asylums: Essays on the Social Situation of Mental Patients and Other Inmates*, Harmondsworth: Penguin.

Griffin, G. (1995) *Feminist Activism in the 1990s*, London: Taylor and Francis.

Hindess, B. (1982) 'Power, interests and the outcomes of struggles', *Sociology* 16(4), 498–511.

Keats, J. (1819) 'Ode to a Nightingale', many anthologies.

Laing, R.D. (1967) *The Politics of Experience and the Bird of Paradise*, Harmondsworth: Penguin.

Lefevre, S. (1996) *Killing Me Softly*, Stockport: Handsell/ACT Publications.

Manic Depression Fellowship (1997) *Inside/Out: A Guide to Self Management*, Kingston-upon-Thames: MDF.

Manic Street Preachers (1994) *The Holy Bible*, disc no. 4774212, Sony Music Entertainment UK Limited

——(1998) *This is my truth tell me yours*, disc no. 4917036, Sony Music Entertainment UK Limited

Melody Maker (1995) 'Manic Depression' and 'From Despair to Where?' 8 April, 29–34.

Mitchell, M. (1998) 'Disciplinary interventions around safer sex', in K. Ellis and D. Hartley (eds) *Social Policy and the Body: Transitions in Corporeal Discourses*, London: Macmillan.

New Musical Express (1994/5).

Norton, K. and Dolan, B. (1996) 'Acting out and the institutional response', in B. Dolan (ed.), *Perpectives On Henderson Hospital*, Sutton, Surrey: Henderson Hospital.

Pembroke, L. (1994) *Self-harm: Perspectives from Personal Experience*, London: Survivors Speak Out.

Plath, S. (1965) *Ariel*, London: Faber and Faber.

Rappaport, J. (1981) 'In praise of paradox: a social policy of empowerment over prevention', in E. Seidman and J. Rappaport (eds), *Redefining Social Problems*, New York: Plenum Press.

Scott James, C. (1990) *Domination and the Arts of Resistance*, New Haven/London: Yale University Press.

Spandler, H. (1996) *Who's Hurting Who? Young People, Self-harm and Suicide*, Manchester: FortySecond Street.

11 Three prisoners' stories
Talking back through autobiography

Steve Morgan

Unlike many of the other groups discussed in this book, prisoners are 'outside' welfare. Prisons are secure and secret places, one of whose functions is to silence the voice of inmates. The acceptable discourse of prisoners is that of remorse and resignation, not explanation or justification. The truths of prison are officially mediated through prison staff and other criminal justice officials. One of the channels of communication open to prisoners after their release is the freedom to tell their stories. The basis of this chapter is a research project to study the corpus of prisoner autobiographies published since 1945 (Morgan, forthcoming). As the project has developed, a number of key areas of interest have emerged: the epistemology of the texts and questions of how they may be read; the authors and the relationship of their lives and identities to the experience of imprisonment; the texts as a means of access to a secret world, normally subject to a high degree of control concerning what can be known about prison and its practices.

The three texts chosen as the focus of the chapter are all written by white men:

* Fletcher, J.W. (1972) *A Menace to Society: My 35 Years in Prison for Stealing £40*
* Leech, M. (1993) *Product of the System: My Life In and Out of Prison*
* Zeno (1968) *Life*

This choice is deliberate, in that men dominate the prison system. Only 4 per cent of prisoners are women. More significantly, the militaristic culture of force and dominance found in prisons is highly gender specific (Sim 1994). In historical terms, each text comes from a different era: the span of publication covers twenty-five years and the period narrated seventy years. The meaning of prison and its practices may thus be interrogated over a substantial period.

The analysis begins by locating the context of the meaning and purpose of prison in orthodox terms with its effect on the credibility of prisoner accounts. This is followed by an overview of the economic and social background of the prison population. The chapter then outlines a theoretical base for the study of autobiography before detailed analysis of the chosen texts and the central themes identified within them.

Prisons and prisoners

The purpose of imprisonment is to exclude the criminal from free society in conditions of security and secrecy, as a means of inflicting a legally authorized measure of punishment equivalent to the pain caused to the victim by the offence. By imprisoning, courts express their outrage against crime and give a warning of the consequences should others seek to commit similar offences. Its secondary function is to place the criminal in physical and moral quarantine so that any criminal acts during sentence may be securely contained within the prison perimeter. If the experience helps to reform or rehabilitate the prisoner, it is a secondary benefit to law-abiding society. Following imprisonment, the act of release requalifies the criminal as a subject fit for reintegration to citizen status (Thomas 1979; Von Hirsch 1976; Bottoms 1983; Walker 1991). This, at least, is the orthodox theory.

This exclusion brings with it significant consequences in loss of civil and legal rights: disqualification from the vote; from access to independent public health care; from any degree of choice in the allocation of a prison, regardless of family circumstances; from the legal safeguards of due process and appeal as these exist outside; from any physical privacy; these are some of the hidden consequences. Total control over access to the physical necessities of daily living (food, clothing, warmth, accommodation, safety, exercise) operates in a system which sets entitlement at a minimum level. It awards all other requirements (letters, visits, home leave, education, sport) as privileges to be earned and thus withdrawn when the prison decides.

The physical separation of prisoners from society is further accentuated by structural and economic divisions and inequalities. In 1991, the first National Prison Survey of a representative sample of 4,000 prisoners was published (Dodd and Hunter 1992). A summary of the main findings (Walmsley *et al.* 1992) forms the basis of the following analysis.

Prisoners were significantly younger than the general population (of those aged 17 or over, 40 per cent were under 25) and predominantly male (only 4 per cent were women). Those describing themselves as black or Asian were heavily over-represented (15 per cent of men, 25 per cent of women compared to less than 6 per cent of the general population). They were more likely to be unskilled or semi-skilled; educationally disadvantaged with higher rates of truancy; unemployed and homeless compared to rates for the general population. For example, 26 per cent had been in care compared to 2 per cent of the population.

The debate concerning the relationship between crime causation and economic disadvantage and unemployment remains contentious (Field 1990; Dickinson 1993). Dickinson has demonstrated a close and striking relationship between rises and falls in property crime and cycles of economic expansion and recession and their effects upon unemployment.

Critical theories of the relationship between economic cycles and the use of imprisonment have been developed by a number of authors (Box and Hale 1982, 1985; Box 1987; Hale 1989; Crow and Simon 1987). These stress the effects of recession upon the ideologies of sentencers and argue that a perception of unemployment as a cause of lawlessness leads to increased imprisonment as a control upon a threatening population. Wilkins (1984) and Pease (1990) both argue that there is a relationship between wide income distribution and the spread of penal measures. The relationship between the economically dispossessed, whose failure is individual, and the profile of the imprisoned, who are individually culpable, becomes a striking association.

Foucault (1977) documents the minutiae of ways in which the prison exercises its power over every aspect of custodial existence. Fifty years before Foucault, an anonymous prisoner described his status:

> Men are animalized here. The governor is responsible to the state to keep the bodies of the men it sends to him for the period stated. I have seen the book marked 'Body Receipt Book'. As soon as we enter, that is what we are, a mere body ... It took me some time to find a fitting condemnation of this well-run machine – clear and regular, but it is that we are treated as bodies without souls. To keep our bodies safe we are counted over 30 times a day – in and out, in and out. You must not do a thing without permission.
>
> (Hobhouse and Brockway 1922: 353)

This loss of agency is accompanied by a loss of credibility. At an academic and practice level, prisoners, as research subjects, have been frequently ignored or marginalized as active participants in explaining offending or evaluating penal measures. The effect of this is to marginalize their contributions as representative of confused and discredited thinking.

Additionally, such accounts are invariably seen as biased. Writing in a period contemporary with two of the texts analysed here, an ex-prisoner takes for granted that:

> Ex-prisoners are not likely to be wholly trustworthy guides to the English prison system. People who go to prison are generally dishonest; or if they are not dishonest, they are likely to be aggrieved for that very reason. In any case, they are not very reliable witnesses.
>
> (Benney 1948: 2)

This common-sense notion of bias and dishonesty as natural characteristics of prisoners is set alongside a promotion of prison officials' truth which is, by its nature, more credible.

So Becker (1967) in his paper *Whose side are we on?* identified a hierarchy of credibility within criminal justice discourse while Cohen and Taylor (1977, 1981) provide the classic account in British criminology of official obstruction of a research project based upon a dialogue with prisoners.

> Our only other 'research technique' was the collaborative writing up of the work. As soon as we had produced a rough description of a particular feature of life in the wing, we would read it to the men and ask for factual and theoretical comments. This exercise also promoted talk in that the men recognized that they were now involved in producing a version of their world which could be transmitted to an outside audience.
>
> (Cohen and Taylor 1977: 72)

In the prison, any talk was subject to codes of minute control and restriction. The authors describe the successful attempt of the Home Office to limit and then cut short their research on the impact of long-term imprisonment, precisely because much of the data was drawn from prisoner accounts. It was uncreditable research and could have no place in any orthodox analysis of the penal system.

To summarize, prisoners represent an unusual and specific social and economic profile which is marked by its typification of social differences and structural inequality. These factors exacerbate the social meaning and experience of imprisonment and its functions of power draining (Mathieson 1990) and exclusion. The stories that prisoners tell of this experience lack official and popular credibility. Autobiography offers a vehicle for an oppositional account to challenge the powerlessness inherent in their public identity and its condemnation.

Public textual discourse and autobiography

The theoretical basis for this chapter is drawn from two different orders of discourse: 'public textual discourse' (Smith 1990) and discourse of autobiography.

Intertextuality is the property of texts to contain explicit and implicit references to or 'snatches of' other existing texts or anticipations of future texts, yet to be produced (Fairclough 1989, 1992). Fairclough argues (1992) that this capacity for interplay between texts is not unlimited or arbitrary since it depends upon relations of power between text producers. While autobiographies are individual stories, many of the texts to which they respond or which they anticipate are produced by more powerful groupings.

These have been named 'official discourse' (Burton and Carlen 1979) or 'public textual discourse' (Smith 1990). Smith stresses the active nature of such texts in 'organizing concerted social action' (ibid.: 121), in this case the action of publicly defining and managing lawbreakers and creating the agenda within which they are to be understood. Such texts (Green and White Papers, legislation, Prison Rules, National Standards for Supervising Offenders in the Community) are the products of specific social relations and institutional processes which organize, govern and supervise offenders and the prison.

Not only do they regulate the lives of offenders and their guards, but in doing so they constitute and reconstitute the nature and characteristics of the offenders. Smith goes on to argue that the institutional language of such texts substitutes 'common sense' and generalized representation for detail, diversity and individuality, producing an orthodox reading of a typical event. This can only be understood by a reader 'in the know' with an insider knowledge of 'who these people really are'.

The dominance of this reconstituted public discourse is reinforced by the tradition and practice of secrecy within prisons. It controls the flow of prison knowledge into the public domain. All discourses of criminal justice are constituted by rhetorical modes of condemnation and resistance which are in turn dominated by metaphors of conflict and warfare: a 'militarized discourse of criminality, built around the metaphor of criminals being "at war" with society, and society having to "mobilize its forces" to "fight them off"' (Fairclough 1992: 130).

Accordingly, credibility is a highly problematic issue. Prisoner autobiography, as a genre, offers a vehicle for the recovery of the detail, diversity and individuality lost in public textual discourse. Plummer (1983: 58) refers to a recovery of '"underdog" perspectives' which challenge '"overdog" perspectives'.

In analysing the discourse of autobiography, it is helpful to use two concepts: context and force in analysis of texts (Fairclough 1992).

Context is created by the interplay between the politics and ideology of the discourse of criminal justice and the social identity of the participants and what Stanley (1993) describes as the social location of authors and readers as constituted in class, race, gender and other determinants of structural inequality.

Force describes the social purpose of the text with its processes of production, distribution and consumption. It presumes an ideal reader. According to Gusdorf (1980: 29), an orthodox autobiography is a product of individualism rooted in the 'cultural awareness of the singularity of each individual life'.

The study of autobiography as discourse and literary form or genre has received renewed interest in the last decade, particularly from feminists. This analysis has emphasized the problems in an orthodox reading: a great life tradition, based upon an exemplary life. This charts the progress of an individual (frequently male, white, middle- or upper-class) from obscurity to fame or from adversity to triumph (Stanley 1992). Such texts are based upon a particular notion of individualism with a privileged vantage point 'above' the other actors in the story and the reader. It consists of: 'the reconstruction on paper of the essential, fundamental person, from a myriad of contemporary, shifting and conflicting views of this event, that relationship, this activity and that achievement' (Stanley 1992: 7).

Gergen and Gergen (1993: 32) reinforce this approach with reference to a 'hero's tale', in which the relationship of writer to reader is constituted as: expert to novice; elder to younger; powerful to powerless.

In contrast feminist readings stress the significance of ordinary lives and the way that the uniqueness of *a* life also 'articulates' (Stanley 1992: 14) with the lives of others. Texts, in this reading, are the result of competing negotiated versions of events but, more than that, certain groups and individuals have to compete with dominant definitions of self and confront these. There are theoretical parallels here to 'public textual discourse' outlined above.

Writing of women's autobiography, Friedman quotes Sheila Rowbottom:

> A woman cannot, Rowbottom argues, experience herself as an entirely unique entity because she is always aware of how she is defined as *woman*, that is, as a member of a group whose identity has been defined by the dominant male culture.
>
> (Friedman 1988: 38, emphasis in original)

The same point in relation to race is made by Du Bois (1903) quoted by Friedman (1988: 40):

> The Negro … is gifted with second sight in this American World – a world which yields him no true self-consciousness but only lets him see himself through the revelation of the other world. It is a peculiar sensation this double consciousness, this sense of always looking at oneself through the eyes of others, of measuring one's soul by the tape of a world that looks on in amused contempt and pity. One ever feels his twoness.
>
> (Du Bois 1903: 30)

These perspectives are echoed in Foucault's writing on the discursive nature of discourse and the creation and use of knowledge as a source of power and a means of subjugation. Foucault, in acknowledging the individual as a 'positive domain of knowledge', creates a means of releasing 'an insurrection of subjugated knowledge' (Foucault 1980: 81).

Such an oppositional perspective in autobiography and discourse has particular relevance to the study of prisoner texts. The authors are members of an outlaw group whose nature and motivations are systematically defined by others through politics, media and other public textual discourse. Garland (1992) has written of the binary and reductive nature of much criminology which:

> operates within an overbearing power structure which makes offenders into problematic objects to be administered, and it is built upon a basic distinction, variously expressed between the criminal and the non-criminal. It tends to generalize, to stereo-

type, to reduce, to objectify and to silence the human beings who fall under its gaze. Only occasionally are we reminded that the objects of the criminological monologue are themselves conscious subjects, who, if only they were allowed to speak, might challenge some of the certainties with which we divide the world into normal and abnormal, right and wrong.

(Garland 1992: 419)

Autobiography offers to prisoners an opportunity to 'challenge some of the certainties' by giving an alternative account of imprisonment and an alternative identity to the author.

Three prisoner autobiographies: critical themes

Analysis of a number of modern prison autobiographies, published in the last fifty years, reveals a theoretical distinction between two groups of texts, both of which are represented in this chapter. For the purpose of analysis within the research, I have labelled these two groups Cons and Straights. These names are chosen first from the prison argot for 'habitual' prisoners and second for a particular group of first offenders characterized by their sense of difference and separation from the Cons.

The texts by Cons give an account of a criminal identity: a life of crime and life in crime. Invariably this history begins with a detailed account of childhood as the source of a relationship to lawbreaking. A particular working-class culture and its interaction with police and other sites of social control (schools or children's homes) is central to this group of texts (McVicar 1974; Boyle 1977; Probyn 1977). For these writers, prison is part of a criminal life and of a coherent narrative development which creates and enhances its specific meaning for the writer. Its cruelty, waste and absurdity are all part of a known and understood lived world.

For the Cons, prison is inevitable, and as the penal system is a battlefield, the prison becomes a major centre of conflict. As each writer narrates and recreates the passage of key stages in a criminal career (reform or approved school, borstal, the adult prison) the sense of shock and disorientation, characteristically portrayed here as the experience of the child or adolescent encountering the system, is rapidly replaced by familiarity and inevitability. This becomes a strong recognition of place within a known culture and network of predictable relationships with both cons and screws. Fletcher (1972) and Leech (1993) are the Cons represented in this chapter.

The Straights are characterized by their refusal to accept a criminal identity. In this group, there is clear evidence that the authors are middle-class, well educated, and that the experience of prison is profoundly alien to their social world. There is a social and cultural difference between the author and other prisoners which is particularly marked in the early stages of prison sentence.

Their relationship to their offence is either to deny it or rationalize it as a mistake, to claim it as political, or implicitly to portray it as a bizarre and unique act unrelated to the identity of the author. Accordingly, imprisonment is an aberration with no coherent links to a past. As a result, the texts narrate only so much of the past as is necessary to put the facts of the sentence in context. There is no account of a personal history or a childhood and only sparse and spasmodic glimpses of any context external to the prison.

The focus of the texts is not the person but the prison as an institution and as an experience with its impact on the self. Zeno (1968) is the representative of this group in the present chapter.

The three autobiographies (Fletcher 1972; Leech 1993; Zeno 1968) will be analysed to examine three key themes: consciousness as resistance to the power of public textual discourse on prisoners; secrecy as the pervasive barrier to prison knowledge; violence within prison and its relationship to styles of masculinity.

The distinction between Cons and Straights is reflected in the different ways in which the authors describe experience. This is most apparent in the section on consciousness but is less marked in the other sections, although its effect upon perspective is invariably present.

Consciousness as resistance

Prisoner autobiographies make a claim to special knowledge, for in an ironic way the writers have access to privileged insider experience of a hidden world. Their claims to the validity of this knowledge are direct and insistent. The address to the reader is explicit and claims, not so much for complete acceptance, but for a reading that is treated as at least as valid as other discourses from prison staff, the media or politicians.

> If an officer so minds he can turn a timid man into a raging beast. So please, dear reader, remember, when you read the papers of violence in prison, that there is usually a prisoner's side to this but you are never given this side to the story.
>
> (Fletcher 1972: 88)

To get an inside picture one must first be convicted, and then of course, anything one has to say is valueless and is treated with the gravest suspicion.

(Zeno 1968: 70)

These claims to credibility, from both a Con and a Straight, are a direct response to the condemnation of prisoners as outlaws. Their negative status is powerfully confirmed in the accounts of confrontations with staff and in prison records. Rituals of degradation inherent in reception to prison, combined with the poverty and squalor of regimes, break down any positive identity.

This is an absolutely silent system. When you speak to an Officer, you turn your back to him and that's the only position you are allowed to speak at any time, with your back to an officer. You are not allowed to look at an officer.

(Fletcher 1972: 34)

This greeting begins a sharply recreated account of reception to Durham prison in the 1930s, a ritual designed to promote the complete degradation of the prisoner. The same rhetoric was used to Mark Leech of entry to Hindley borstal in 1974. 'Address every member of staff as Sir, double when you're told to double, your cell is to be left clean and tidy – no shit in the piss-pots – and if you're looking for a pleasant time here, forget it' (Leech 1993: 36).

The social practices of penal institutions are not particularly imaginative but they are at least consistent.

Each of the three authors responds to the ascribed identity differently. Bill Fletcher withdraws into himself as the passive recipient of discipline through self-isolation and doing his bird. His account of a childhood spent in abusive and violent reform schools from the age of 6 and rejection by his family create a basis for a life of self-reliance through petty delinquency and perpetual custody.

Prison taught me what real terror is, the terror of being helpless when people hate you, what it is to be at the mercy of sadism, because they play with men at their mercy in prison. I do not think I will ever really get over that feeling of terror knowing what the authorities could do to a man like me, and can still do to this day, because with a record you are never out of their clutches.

(Fletcher 1972: 10)

His resistance is not through active opposition but inside the head: 'I managed to follow my own path, leaving the screws alone and they left me alone but everything happened around me' (Fletcher 1972: 59).

Fletcher served a total of 35 years, including 8 years from 1961 for the theft of ten shillings: 'to protect society from people like you' (ibid.: 97). Yet he never identifies himself as a criminal.

> The reason I have never become a criminal in all my years in prison is because I have seen what real crime can do to people … and I am not a criminal because to be a criminal you must have a vicious mind and have no regard for other people and you do not believe in God.
>
> (ibid.: 135)

He follows the prisoner code of nonco-operation with prison staff but is not involved in violence or direct subversion of the system. He makes no relationship with fellow prisoners. At one point he refuses to obey an order to work and completes the final two and a half years of his sentence in solitary confinement. The result is a man who becomes completely institutionalized and terrified of life outside the prison.

> The first thing that gets you is the noise and the movement of traffic. Within an hour you are a nervous wreck for the pace of life is like nothing you have experienced inside, where all is quiet and you lead a monastic life with everything moving slowly along, no noise, no hurry and scurry. You are in a crowd of people, yet you are lonely, lost and bewildered. You are afraid to go even into a shop for you feel everyone is looking at your antics.
>
> (ibid.: 82)

All meaningful contacts with an identity other than that of prisoner are lost, as positive links to family had been broken as a young man. Indeed, 'The fact that I had no family ties and therefore no outside worries I am sure is the only reason I did not go insane through all the time I served' (ibid.: 103).

Mark Leech describes a very similar account of early experiences in remand homes and approved schools where violence and sexual abuse from staff and other boys was routine. The result of this treatment was the internalization of a powerful hatred, not only of any form of authority but also of himself. At 19:

I was a complete arsehole, out to do as much damage as I could and would not stand anyone being in control of me. I hated authority in all its guises. I was selfish beyond belief and did not have many friends; those I had never remained around for long and I don't blame them – I hated me too.

(Leech 1993: 47)

In his case, passivity gave way to continuing and active violent and non-violent resistance. The violence will be discussed in the next section, but an alternative and more productive strategy emerged through legal studies and the use of petitions and legal action to challenge the prison system within the courts.

In Wormwood Scrubs, the education department offered the opportunity to study law.

I enrolled and was at once captivated by the subject. I studied every single day and long into the nights. As the education officer put it, 'Mark, if you want to play the game and fight the system, you first have to learn the rules.'

(Leech 1993: 53–4)

This strategy led to significant victories regarding abuses of due process and natural justice in Boards of Visitors' hearings.

The turning point came with his transfer to the 'therapeutic' regime at Grendon Underwood. The irony of Grendon is that, although the treatment regime pathologizes the prisoner in that all responsibility for change is seen to rest in attitude changes in the individual, the method used turns some aspects of the prison power structure and practices on their head.

The confrontational and militaristic culture which normally denies prisoners any degree of autonomy and denies open expression of frustration or criticism towards staff was replaced by a culture of assertive challenges. Some officers found this role and power reversal exceptionally difficult.

'Yes, I want to change my life, but I don't need the nutters which this place contains to enable me to do it.' He smiled. 'When I came here, I too found it fucking difficult to come to terms with. All my service had been spent in the system and this place turns that on its head ... but after a while, when you start to see the good that this place can do – and yes it takes hard work – then you begin to realize what the penal system should really be about, not banging prisoners up in strip cells and kicking all kinds of shit out of them.' I respected his honesty.

(ibid.: 130)

In Grendon, the author is able to confront his anger and aggression and its roots in physical and sexual abuse. Crucial, also, is the acknowledgement of his own sexuality as a gay man, long acknowledged but never publicized within the homophobic but ambiguous prejudices of the male prison system. The support of the parents of another prisoner had given him a family focus beyond the prison.

The personal success involved in these changes is frustrated when Grendon has to be closed and the wing is transferred to Leicester, where opposition from the orthodox system is strong. During this period he begins to write plays and journalism and discover an alternative identity. Transfer to an open prison takes him close to release, when the shock of discovery of his HIV status leads to absconding, further offences and re-imprisonment as the text ends.

In contrast, Zeno, as a Straight, writes from a different consciousness. His *nom de plume*, the leading Greek stoic philosopher, makes a statement of acceptance and resignation in the face of the inevitable. The title both reflects the mandatory sentence for murder and is an ironic comment upon the boundaries of his existence in prison. There is a strong sense of initial separateness from 'real' criminals, a superiority by class and education.

> While on remand, I have seen something of the men with whom I am to spend the indeterminate number of years which lie ahead of me, and I am not particularly impressed one way or the other. Those I have met seem very commonplace, rather below the average in intelligence, but that is what one would expect. One of the screws has already told me that I cannot hold the Prison Commissioners responsible for the company I have to keep in prison.
>
> (Zeno 1968: 12)

His separate status is reflected in his social class and education and in the staff recognition of lifers as exceptional prisoners.

Whereas the two Cons write with increasingly dismissive familiarity of their known world, Zeno, as an outsider, draws the reader into a shared sense of shock at the realities of an unknown world. As he meets prison conditions, the reader is invited to share in the naivety of his ignorance.

I have heard the humiliating abuse, the foul-mouthed obscenities, the defiant replies, the whimpering acceptance, the bang of doors, the rattle of keys, the slop of empty chamber pots … On the faces of some of the screws an animal brutality, a shallow-eyed insensitivity that is hard to imagine as being wholly human … on the faces of a few of them, a very few, traces of occasional compassion.

(ibid.: 19)

He describes the gradual process of his conversion to a new consciousness:

After a year I have taken sides. At no time would I have considered joining the enemy, but in the early days I had hoped that at least I could stand apart as an impartial observer … In my six months in the Scrubs I have become conscious of other factors, sickened by the uselessness of our existence, shocked by the combination of hypocrisy and dishonesty in those who dictate the details of our daily lives. I find I think less and less about the enormity of my offence. They have forced out of my mind the nagging memory of the man I killed. It is as if the sharp pain of a bad tooth, by its persistence, has eliminated the dull ache of a cancer.

(ibid.: 52)

As his sentence (nine years in custody) passes, his re-education and that of the reader continues and sympathy passes much more explicitly to the prisoners. Although Zeno's experience and class position clearly distance him from aspects of the prison culture and enable him to obtain professional employment on release within a known and secure world, there remains a new sense of alienation from that world. He appears almost stateless. What has changed is the loss of a secure sense of place, of the capacity for intimacy and of belief in a fair and equitable justice system.

Secrecy

Secrecy, in its many forms, is a pervasive and dominant influence upon every aspect of prison life. It is an important strategy in the management of power relations. It attempts to control knowledge by the supervision of all activity and communication. There are official and unofficial codes of who may talk to whom and in what circumstances, and what is permissible to be said. The effects of secrecy are active and are experienced at two levels in the prison.

These are, first, the effects of the physical and human barriers (the wall and staff surveillance) and second, through the role of secrecy in human relations between prisoners and staff.

The wall or fence is the architectural barrier enforcing containment and preventing access to the unauthorized. Its symbolic nature is expressed in its massive and imposing architecture whose explicit purpose was to create foreboding and dread in the mind of the Straight outsider. 'The prison wall was built of blocks of granite or some other similar stone. It is lowering and oppressive, and seems to exude a grey, almost invisible cloud of depression' (Zeno 1968: 12).

The physical barrier is strengthened by staff surveillance: the censorship of communications, letters and visits; the physical searching (rub downs and internal body searches and of the 'private' space of the cell and personal possessions). All communication into and out of the prison is governed by the intricacies of prison rules and the Official Secrets Act (Cohen and Taylor 1976).

> Despite what the Home Office says about having abandoned censorship of mail, all letters to and from the prisoner – with the sole exception of letters covered by legal privilege – are routinely censored; the Home Office, when it redrafted the rules following the Woolf report in 1990, purposely left themselves with a residual power of censorship.
>
> (Leech 1993: 41)

Prisoners are not entitled to unofficial communication. All official communication is conducted through complex stages of procedure. Any failure to follow these may lead to disqualification of the process and a return to the beginning of the procedure. Any letter containing any form of 'allegation' criticizing the prison may be required to be rewritten if 'the allegations had not been previously ventilated through the complaints procedure' (ibid.: 85).

The autobiographies, from both Straight and Con perspectives, all reveal the extent of the waste, absurdity and general inefficiency hidden by official secrecy.

> It's all a phoney game and we are the pawns ... A satisfactory image of something being done must be presented to the public, and be supported by figures convincing enough to satisfy a not too thorough inspection, and if enquiries are pushed beyond a certain point they can always be blocked or diverted into other channels.
>
> (Zeno 1968: 69)

This prevents any possibility of change because failings and weaknesses cannot be acknowledged and, therefore, cannot be addressed.

The second sphere in which secrecy plays a dominant role is the construction of the prison record. This dossier is compiled upon the prisoner, reconstructing the new identity both from materials known to the prisoner (police record, probation report) as well as from a mass of unknown and uncheckable observations, recorded by staff and hidden from the subject. This is starkly emphasized when Mark Leech meets an officer in Grendon.

> He asked me about my past and I noticed throughout our conversation he did not take notes; prison officers *always* take notes, either as a result of their inability to recall basic facts or the system's need for raw data.
>
> (Leech 1993: 125, original emphasis)

This creation is aided by the panoptic character of the prison in which all activity is potentially subject to the gaze of staff, from the most public areas (workshops, exercise) to the most private (bathing and defecation). If suspected of hiding contraband, the prisoner may be searched internally. Privacy in prison is non-existent.

Prisoners' resistance to this panoptic gaze is primarily mounted via the inmate code of secrecy ('no grassing to screws') which dominates prisoner–staff relations. All three authors recognize and follow this, despite their distinct differences in orientation to the experience of prison. The Straight, Zeno, explains its internal logic:

> To many people, this refusal to inform on other men must seem a distorted and perverted form of loyalty, particularly when violence and injury go unpunished, perhaps unchecked, as a direct result of silence, but it is not as simple as it appears. We are all aware, some consciously, some unconsciously, that once the habit of informing starts, there will be no end to it.
>
> (Zeno 1968: 155)

Parallel to the code of prisoner secrecy, there exists an identical, if less apparent, staff code. This maintains that as prisoners are, by their very nature, untrustworthy and uncredible, their explanation or evidence in any conflict with staff can never be believed.

Zeno shares the loss of his own naivety with the reader, reflecting on one of his fellow prisoners:

Looking at his face I feel suddenly an empathetic understanding of his view of a world in which the only people who believe a particular truth which is important to him are others like himself, helpless men, mostly inarticulate, and all of them criminals whose word is valueless. He doesn't count the others who know the truth, the screws who close ranks and lie to protect themselves and each other. In a court the man who is a thief or guilty of violence must always be a liar. The prison officer and policeman who are not criminals must always be men of truth and integrity.

(ibid.: 58)

Whatever staff may 'know' about an incident which could favour a prisoner's case, it must remain a secret from the prisoner. This is a source of very considerable power in disciplinary proceedings when a prisoner is reported for any breach of prison rules. 'Officers at Wormwood Scrubs do not tell lies. If they tell me you have been riding a motor-bike around the fucking exercise yard, then I want to know where you got the petrol' (Leech 1993: 51).

Although almost certainly apocryphal, this style of confrontation and the rigidity of these two codes creates a culture in which there can be only two 'truths' in opposition, in which the hierarchy of credibility must favour the staff.

It is the challenge to this confrontation, inherent in the regime at Grendon, which is so immediately striking and disturbing to Mark Leech. The idea that prisoners must be directly honest to each other and to staff, may have to 'inform' upon each other, and that staff may admit their fault, reverses the orthodox discourse of prison relations.

Not only is this difficult for prisoners, it is a focus of deep hostility from staff outside the groups and in other prisons. The Grendon system of challenging the sterility and rigidity of prisoner–officer relations offers alternative space for acknowledgement of prisoner credibility. As with the Special Unit at Barlinnie (Boyle 1977) in Scotland, Grendon is the only other prison to introduce such an approach with serious and dangerous prisoners in England and Wales on a consistent and continuing basis. It has not been extended and the Barlinnie unit has closed.

Violence

The practice of secrecy is an important strategy in the concealment of the role and levels of violence in men's prisons. Prisoner autobiographies clarify the fact that violence is endemic as a key manifestation of a culture of masculine dominance, critical to the functioning of the prison. In a recent paper, Sim (1994) focuses on the role of violent masculinity in prison and its position as the basis of power relations. Force and the threat of force lie behind many of the everyday interactions between staff and prisoners and among prisoners themselves.

Both Bill Fletcher and Mark Leech, as Cons, describe its emergence in the earliest stages of their criminal careers. Sexual and physical abuse and bullying in reform and approved schools by staff and by older stronger boys is endemic. Its existence is not just casual but an integral part of the disciplinary practices of the school, in which staff 'delegate' aspects of control to other boys. Fletcher refers to the 'sadism, cruelty and real hatred' (Fletcher 1972: 9) engendered in borstal. His initiation to Durham prison, described earlier, emphasizes the role of force in confirming the subjugated identity of all prisoners. Violent gangs in Portland borstal and later in Dartmoor are clear examples of a culture in which 'rep' and being 'a bit tasty' are essential attributes of identity and survival in a hierarchy built upon physical dominance.

Mark Leech describes how 'I have been brutalized and how I, in return, have brutalized others' (Leech 1993: 13). The history of the early part of his prison career was dominated by consistent and systematic violent resistance. This included attacks upon other prisoners, upon prison staff, including smearing his own faeces in the face of Dartmoor's governor. The result was heavy loss of remission and retaliatory beatings by prison staff in punishment cells, the most secret and separate part of any prison, whose violence and physical repression is hidden from the remainder of the institution. His description of this process emphasizes the way in which the culture of force can, in its most mundane as well as its most extreme forms, create an environment in which no space exists for alternative responses.

All three authors emphasize its effect upon the better instincts of both prisoners and officers.

> Underneath all the bullshit and shouting – which is part of any prison officer's make-up – I found a kind and caring man who really wanted to help but was prevented from doing so by the constraints of the system within which he operated.
>
> (Leech 1993: 36)

> I know he is aware of things he can never admit to me that he knows. Before he turns back to me, he sighs visibly, and I can only guess at the conflicting thoughts and emotions which bring on the

sigh. Weariness under the impossible task he shoulders, sadness at
the almost complete lack of trust placed in him and his fellows by
us.

(Zeno 1968: 113–14)

As a Straight, Zeno has a different relationship to the place of
violence within the prison. Early in the sentence he is sceptical, an
'unbiased' observer, he remains completely uninvolved in any incidents.
Yet his low-key accounts of fights, attacks and staff responses emphasize their systematic nature through the very quality of understatement
within the text. He notes the effect of the restriction of the compulsory
periods of free association on the wing in Wormwood Scrubs: 'Since
men are no longer forced to associate with each other in large
numbers, three-quarters of the violence, fighting and bloodshed no
longer occurs' (Zeno 1968: 155).

This hegemony of force, although instituted and largely controlled
by staff, traps them as effectively as it dominates the lives of those they
lock up. But, as Sim (1994) emphasizes, this culture of masculinity is
not peculiar to prisons but is endemic in all male-dominated institutions (armed forces, male public schools, the police) and is only an
extreme form of the dominance enjoyed by men in all major social
institutions.

Sim argues that the normalization and routinization of physical
domination compromises any potential for change. As Bill Fletcher
shows, fear is a constant reality for many prisoners. Only a minority of
prisoners are violent or hard men. Mark Leech, in the midst of his
own violent resistance, can reach out to the plight of a friend who had
been refused parole (and who subsequently hanged himself).

I put my arm around the man who was probably the kindest and
gentlest man I had ever known, and as he cried out his pain I
could only feel hatred for the inhumane life sentence system which
caused such heartache and anguish. There were no explanations
for why he had not been given a release date, nothing to soften the
blow or help him to be more prepared to present his case next
time.

(Leech 1993: 101)

The regime at Grendon and to a lesser degree that at Maidstone
prison are the only two examples of attempts to create change.
Grendon's emphasis upon breaking down the culture of confrontation
only existed within part of that prison. Other wings maintained a more

orthodox regime. Hostility to the special unit at Barlinnie caused its eventual closure.

Conclusion

These authors make a direct claim for the validity of their accounts, based upon a specific experience from a particular standpoint, to be accepted as their truth. Despite their differences in history and perspective, the Cons and the Straight are ultimately united in a common critique of prison, based upon their experiences. The texts are only a small part of a much wider system of genres, all contributing to the discourse of the prison and of criminal justice. The elements in this discourse were earlier characterized by a strong emphasis upon modes of condemnation and resistance. These texts contain oppositional voices.

The central strategy in exercising power and control within the prison has been secrecy. The wall and the Official Secrets Act together have attempted to create an impermeable barrier to such voices. Official discourse declares that offenders' accounts are incomplete and partial or simply untrue, and claims security as the main reason for the denial of an alternative account. So, with its allies in the media, it seeks to control what can be said about prisons.

The squalor and poverty of physical conditions is starkly identified. The rigidity and confrontation of prisoner–officer relations invariably drags the behaviour of each down to a common denominator of pettiness, sterility and force. Any space for an alternative is stifled. There is ample evidence of the replication and inflation of the worst abuses of power by physical dominance in the world beyond the prison. The potential for corruption, waste and real danger are emphasized by detail in the texts. The lost opportunities for any real rehabilitation outweigh the small number of positive experiments.

This has major implications for those who work with prisoners and for those who carry out research in prisons. Without the voice of the prisoners being heard, understanding of the prison as a social institution and of its practices will be partial and incomplete. This denial of credibility has also been strengthened by the growing dominance, in the last ten years, of the use of cognitive behavioural methods in work with offenders in the community (Morgan 1995). These methods, characterized by the 'What Works' movement (McGuire 1995) are based upon a central conception of lawbreaking as a product of faulty thinking and poor development of cognitive reasoning. Protagonists argue that it is the task of those who work with offenders to use programmes based upon behavioural methods to modify and change these distorted belief systems. This chapter asserts that such an analysis, if extended to any testimony by offenders, is ideological and misplaced and ultimately counter-productive.

The irony is that prisons are only governable with significant co-operation from those they house. Denial of the validity of their accounts, refusal to acknowledge the part played by poverty and its associated social exclusions and inequalities, is ultimately self-defeating. Continuation of the current prison culture of dominance by force can only lead to its extension and intensification.

Any final conclusion on reading prisoner autobiography leaves the stark impression of a dysfunctional system that is both wasteful and deeply destructive to all those whose lives it controls. In her commentary upon the stories of four women prisoners, Carlen *et al.* (1985: 182–3) summarize the functions of women's imprisonment. Its purpose is to 'Discipline, Infantilize, Feminize, Medicalize and Domesticize'.

Study of these three texts provides evidence for an alternative summary of functions, particularly for male prisons: to anatomize, ritualize, brutalize, criminalize and institutionalize.

References

Becker, H.S. (1967) 'Whose side are we on?', *Social Problems*, 14, 239–47.
Benney, M. (1948) *Gaol Delivery*, London: Longman, Green and Co.
Bottoms, A.E. (1983) 'Neglected features of contemporary penal systems', in D. Garland and P. Young (eds), *The Power to Punish: Contemporary Penalty and Social Analysis*, London: Heinemann.
Box, S. (1987) *Recession, Crime and Punishment*, London: Macmillan.
Box, S. and Hale, C. (1982) 'Economic crisis and the rising prisoner population in England and Wales', *Crime and Social Justice*, 17, 20–3.
——(1985) 'Unemployment, imprisonment and prison overcrowding', *Contemporary Crises*, 9, 208–29.
Boyle, J. (1977) *A Sense of Freedom*, London: Pan Books.
Burton, F. and Carlen, P. (1979) *Official Discourse*, London: Routledge and Kegan Paul.
Carlen, P., Hicks, J., O'Dwyer, J., Christina, D. and Tchaikovsky, C. (1985) *Criminal Women: Autobiographical Accounts*, London: Polity Press.
Cohen, S. and Taylor, L. (1976) *Prison Secrets*, London: National Council for Civil Liberties, Radical Alternatives to Prison.
——(1977) 'Talking about prison blues', in C. Bell and H. Newby (eds), *Doing Sociological Research*, London: George Allen and Unwin.
——(1981) [1972] *Psychological Survival: The Experience of Longterm Imprisonment*, (second edition) Harmondsworth: Penguin.

Crow, I. and Simon, F. (1987) *Unemployment and Magistrates Courts*, London: Nacro.

Dickinson, D. (1993) *Crime and Unemployment*, Cambridge: Cambridge University Press.

Dodd, T. and Hunter, P. (1992) *The National Prison Survey, 1991*, London: HMSO.

Du Bois, W.E.B. (1968) [1903] 'The Souls of Black Folk', in A. Chapman (ed.), *Black Voices: An Anthology of Afro-American Literature*, New York: New American Library.

Fairclough, N. (1989) *Language and Power*, London, New York: Longman.

——(1992) *Discourse and Social Change*, London: Polity Press.

Field, S. (1990) *Trends in Crime and their Interpretation: A Study in Postwar England and Wales*, Home Office Research Study no. 119, London: HMSO.

Fletcher, J.W. (1972) *A Menace to Society: My 35 Years in Prison – for Stealing £40*, London: Paul Elek Books.

Foucault, M. (1977) *Discipline and Punish: The Birth of the Prison*, Harmondsworth: Penguin.

——(1980) 'Prison talk', in C. Gordon (ed.), *Power/Knowledge: Selected Interviews and Other Writings, 1977–84*, London: Routledge.

Friedman, S.S. (1988) 'Women's autobiographical selves: theory and practice', in S. Benstock (ed.), *The Private Self: Theory and Practice of Women's Autobiographical Writings*, London: Routledge.

Garland, D. (1992) 'Criminological knowledge and its relation to power: Foucault's genealogy and criminology today', *British Journal of Criminology*, 32, 403–22.

Gergen, M.M. and Gergen, K.J. (1993) 'Autobiographies and the shaping of gendered lives', in N. Coupland and J.F. Nussbaum (eds) *Discourse and Lifespan Identity*, New York: Sage.

Gusdorf, G. (1980) [1956] 'Conditions and limits of autobiography', translated by J. Olney, in J. Olney (ed.), *Autobiography: Essays Theoretical and Critical*, Princeton: University of Princeton Press, 28–48.

Hale, C. (1989) 'Economy, punishment and imprisonment', *Contemporary Crises*, 13, 327–49.

Hobhouse, S. and Brockway, F. (1922) *English Prisons Today*, London: Prison System Enquiry Committee.

Leech, M. (1993) *Product of the System: My Life in and out of Prison*, London: Gollancz.

McGuire, J. (ed.) (1995) *What Works: Reducing Reoffending. Guidelines from Research and Practice*. London, New York: John Wiley and Sons.

McVicar, J. (1974) *McVicar by Himself*, edited with an introduction by Goronwy Rees, London: Pan Books.

Mathieson, T. (1990) *Prison on Trial*, London: Sage.

Morgan, S. (1995) *Hearing Offenders: Uncredited Voices in Probation Research and Evaluation*, Manchester: Manchester Metropolitan University.

——(1999) 'Prison lives: critical issues in reading prisoner autobiography', *The Howard Journal of Criminal Justice*, 38, 328–340.

Pease, K. (1990) 'Punishment demand and punishment numbers', in D. Gottfriedson and R. Clarke (eds), *Policy and Theory in Criminal Justice*, Aldershot: Avebury.

Plummer, K. (1983) *Documents of Life: An Introduction to the Problems and Literature of a Humanistic Method*, London: Unwin Hyman.

Probyn, W. (1977) *Angel Face: The Making of a Criminal*, London: Allen and Unwin.

Sim, J. (1994) 'Tougher than the rest: men in prison', in T. Newburn and E.A. Stanko (eds), *Just Boys Doing Business*, London: Routledge.

Smith, D. (1990) *Texts, Facts and Femininity*, London, New York: Routledge.

Stanley, L. (1992) *The Auto/biographical I: The Theory and Practice of Feminist Autobiography*, Manchester: Manchester University Press.

——(1993) 'On autobiography in sociology', *Sociology*, 27, 41–52.

Thomas, D.A. (1979) *Principles of Sentencing: The Sentencing Policies of the Court of Appeal Criminal Division* (second edition), London: Heinemann.

Von Hirsch, A. (1976) *Doing Justice: The Choice of Punishments*, Report of the Committee for the Study of Incarceration, New York: Hill and Wang.

Walker, N. (1991) *Why Punish?*, Oxford: Oxford University Press.

Walmsley, R., Howard, L. and White, S. (1992) *The National Prison Survey: Main Findings*, Home Office Research Study no. 128, London: HMSO.

Wilkins, L. (1984) *Consumerist Criminology*, Aldershot: Gower.

Zeno (1968) *Life*, London: Macmillan.

12 In or out?

How lesbians negotiate and experience coming out

Helen Williamson

When I chose to research how lesbians deal with coming out, I was faced with an irony. In putting my name to this chapter I am 'outing' myself to people who do not know I am a lesbian. I am often asked 'what is your work about?' and so I live my own individual experience of coming out. Rising anxiety and unwillingness to be dishonest combine with fear of rejection. Much of my life's energy has gone into negotiating coming out to family, friends, work colleagues and others. What do I risk if I do, or do not, come out? Having struggled with a lack of confidence and fear of isolation, particularly in my adolescent years, I now have a strong network of friends, a supportive family, a choice of job where I can 'be myself' – but I can still experience feelings of inadequacy and self-deprecation. Why?

Lesbian sexuality and the problem of coming out are rarely acknowledged, and most people are unaware of how unrelenting the question of disclosure can be. In discussions about oppression, sexuality is ignored or greeted with embarrassed indifference or hostility. In social work training I discovered similar degrees of homophobia among students as one might find elsewhere, and some teaching reflected ignorance about heterosexism. Coming out in this unsafe environment, which I felt I needed to do, was extremely stressful. My contact with qualified social workers has reinforced these concerns.

Lesbian sexuality is a complex subject which 'has never reached the heady heights of respectability' (Cosis-Brown 1998: 24). Heterosexuality is 'compulsory in its insistent taken for grantedness' (Epstein and Johnson, 1994: 198) and it is this that gives heterosexuality its power. The research I undertook (Williamson 1997) was an attempt to give both myself and the women I interviewed a *voice*, to confront the distortion of experience and silencing faced by many lesbians. However, the ambition to give a voice to other lesbians is complex. In attempting to empower I would be part of a power process, and what the women said would be mediated by me. Would I be appropriating their voice(s) and rendering them powerless in some way? In attempting to minimize these effects I located the methods and analysis within the traditions of feminist and lesbian and gay emancipatory research (Graham 1993; Carabine 1996; Hicks and McDermott 1999).

This chapter examines commonly held beliefs that lesbians 'ram the issue down our throats', or make a fuss about nothing. It aims to show how deeply our lives are affected and to draw out the implications for social work. It describes experiences of coming out and complexities in the ways coming out is negotiated. First, it is important to define homophobia and heterosexism because they impact on the subject of coming out.

Homophobia

Card (1995) defines homophobia as a fear and a hatred and contempt for people sexually and emotionally attracted to the same sex. Lesbians are often perceived as being perverted and abnormal. Its origin is complex but Lorde (1985: 5) places it in context: 'We have been taught to fear all difference'.

Heterosexism

Heterosexism is a belief in the superiority of heterosexuality over homosexuality (Lorde 1985). Markowe (1996) adds that it encompasses inflexible gender role expectations of women and notions of normality. Lesbians are seen as a threat to the status quo because they defy both expected sexuality and gender roles, and many lesbians fear being too visible. Lesbian mothers, for example, 'are forced to be silent when the weight of society ... and the family come together' (Brosnan 1996: 25).

Coming out is negotiated in the context of widespread homophobia and heterosexism, perpetuated, as with other forms of oppression, through the education system, the media, religion and other institutional practices. Why, then, bother to contemplate coming out at all, given the level of stress? Rakusen's (1989: 203) reply is: 'Heterosexuals can hold hands in public, go anywhere together, be welcomed as a couple by their families and at religious services, celebrate their relationships openly ... lesbians can take none of these things for granted.'

Heterosexuality is everywhere affirmed. Television, advertising, newspapers, are all targeted towards the heterosexual majority (Byrne and Larkin 1994). Lesbians will often only receive acknowledgement of their existence – often in pathological ways – if they register their presence and voice their needs. Weeks (1987: 31) summarizes this point well: heterosexuality is 'the great unsaid of our sexual culture'. It is not necessary to state 'I am heterosexual' because it is already assumed.

Coming out

The term implies 'coming out of the closet', out of hiding. 'Coming out is the process of accepting yourself as a lesbian and figuring out how open you want to be about your sexual orientation' (Outright 1991: 4). The 'closet' is a heterosexual construction – an attempt to make us silent and invisible. There are no rules about how best to come out, but it can often occur in stages: first coming out to ourselves: then coming out to other lesbians or those we feel will be accepting: finally coming out to our family or workmates (Lovell 1995). As Hall (1993) says, coming out is a continuous process of complex decision-making, sometimes planned, sometimes occurring spontaneously. The need for the choice is unrelenting and arises when we encounter a new person, new situation or new job. It also occurs 'in print, public lectures, interviews, conversations, even parades ... usually it is less exhibitionist (although it raises more eyebrows) than common heterosexual displays of marriage' (Card 1995: 204).

It may also have historic or political consequences, as in the case of Oscar Wilde which contributed to changes in the law for gay men, or the events of Stonewall, resulting in an increasingly assertive gay and lesbian community. It can also be achieved through association with groups campaigning for civil and social rights (Signorile 1995; Weeks 1990). Coming out is fundamentally about having a sense of choice and control (Rich 1980). The literature makes clear the diversity of background and age among lesbians. Some have known for years about their sexuality, some not until much later in life. Some spend years in confusion and isolation, some come out early and link into support networks that help cushion the stress of coming out. Some marry because of family expectations, and this is especially true for older women. Where one lives also has an influence on coming out, it being generally harder in small or rural communities. Often lesbian identities are hidden unless disclosed, 'this in effect hides or masks both their lesbian identities and the specificity of that oppression' (Appleby 1994: 28). When sexuality *is* disclosed, we may be faced with powerful stigmatization and negative stereotypes of lesbians as aggressive man-haters. The word 'lesbian' is commonly used as an insult – in coming out we have to identify ourselves as 'belonging' to this nega-tively perceived group.

It is clear from the literature that the negotiation of coming out, with all its complexities, the reactions of family, friends and work colleagues, has played a central part in the lives of many lesbians, a constant presence unknown to heterosexuals. Coming out can evoke both negative and positive experiences. Feelings of rejection, hostility and isolation may be experienced alongside feelings of affirmation and the chance to meet other lesbians as friends and maybe as lovers.

Research done by Marland Hitchcock and Skodal Wilson (1992) on lesbian disclosure to health care professionals details stages of antici-pation, imagined outcomes and 'sussing out', through verbal and non-verbal cues such as literature in the waiting room, whether written information assumes heterosexuality, how health professionals dress and relate to us. Lesbians consider many such factors before they decide to come out.

Markowe (1996) makes the point that lesbianism and heterosexu-ality are social constructs – they are not 'natural', pre-given states of being, but vary geographically, historically and culturally. In most countries coming out is contemplated within a context of inflexible gender roles, concepts of 'normality' and 'abnormality', sexism and inequality of power between lesbians and heterosexuals. The notion of coming out would not exist in a culture that valued difference.

Apart from lesbian testimonies or life stories, which by their nature allow for self-identification (age, race, etc.), few studies deal adequately with the interplay of other oppressions on the coming-out process, especially race and disability. Some authors admit that this aspect is missing from their research but do not acknowledge that this neces-sarily makes it representative particularly of white, able-bodied and often younger lesbians. Some research does address disability (Appleby 1994) and older lesbians (Neild and Pearson 1992), describing stigma and invisibility. Both disabled and older lesbians (not mutually exclu-sive) are often presumed to have no sexuality. Some disabled lesbians fear loss of support because they have to rely heavily on significant others. Some women feel their disability makes them less able to protect themselves against potential aggression. However, there is little looking at coming out in holistic ways related to, for example, age, race, disability and motherhood. Lesbians *are* white, black, disabled, able-bodied, old and young. While certain experiences are common, the understanding of other oppressions can modify our approaches to coming out.

Choosing a method

My objective as a researcher, to give others a voice/to represent the views of others as faithfully as I could, is placed firmly within the context of common *and* diverse experience, an attempt to speak on 'behalf' of others without appropriating and misrepresenting their views. There has been much discussion of 'representing the other' in feminist research (e.g. Mohanty 1991; Yeatman 1993; Truman 1994), and it continues to be a topic of ongoing debate. Central to any attempt to work in emancipatory ways is a recognition of the researcher's own implication in power and the importance of constantly interrogating one's behaviour in the process. Part of this interrogation is the recognition that for some lesbians 'giving a voice' means empowerment through remaining silent. I return to this later.

The question was, how could I give *myself* a voice, yet present, with minimum displacement, the views and experiences of the women I interviewed? I could only do so with an awareness of the diversity that exists among lesbians, and an acknowledgement of my power as researcher within this. I would not be an advocate, but would use my research to highlight the complexities of coming out and the impact of other oppressions on this. Inevitably I would choose what emphasis to place on the results but, by using minimal interpretation, I could allow participants to speak for themselves *as much as possible*, enabling readers to draw their own conclusions from the data. The experience was contradictory for me. Being a lesbian myself resulted in gaining trust and representing other lesbians directly. At the same time, research into sexuality carries a stigma for the researcher (Kitzinger 1987; Signorile 1995), in addition to my being 'outed', with its familiar positive and negative ramifications.

I tape-recorded in-depth interviews with fifteen lesbians aged 15–72, asking them to self-identify their race/ethnicity, disability and class. Pseudonyms were used to protect anonymity. Table 12.1 shows the characteristics of the women interviewed. Inevitably, the women who are heard here are those prepared to be interviewed. I have organized their responses around a number of typical situations with minimal comment from me.

Experiencing coming out

Individuals deal with the issue of coming out very differently, developing a range of strategies. At times we feel comfortable stating our sexuality, at other times we choose *not* to be heard because it does not

Table 12.1   Characteristics of the women interviewed

Name	Age	Race	Class	Disability	Children	Employment status
Lin	15	Chinese born in England	Working class	No	0	At school
Diane	24	White English	Working class	No	0	Employed
Joanne	26	African-Caribbean	Working class	No	0	'Officially' unemployed
Tracy	29	Jewish	Middle class	No	0	Unemployed
Asantewaa	30	African	Working class	No	2	Employed
Pauline	32	White British	Working class	No	0	Employed
Julie	34	White English	Working class	No	0	Employed
Kath	34	British Asian	Working class	No	0	Self-employed
Angela	37	Internationalist	Below middle	Yes	0	Self-employed
Anne	42	White English	Classless	No	6	Employed
Sue	49	White English	Working Class	Yes	2	Receiving disability benefits
Geeta	54	Indian	Working Class	No	0	Employed
Elsa	54	White Scottish	Lower Middle	Yes	2	Receiving disability benefits
Trish	54	White Irish	Working Class	No	4	Self-employed
Ruth	72	White English	Classless	Yes	2	Retired

feel safe or relevant. Strategies develop according to our perceptions of each situation, the people involved, possible outcomes, and the particular circumstances. This process is a significant part of daily life for many of the lesbians I interviewed. Below are typical responses to situations confronted on a daily basis.

How do we judge how people might react?

> Usually within five minutes of meeting someone you more or less know if ... their response would be appropriate.
>
> (Angela)

> How they vote, where they live, what their attitudes are to other minorities.
>
> (Diane)

> I'm not out to my children ... I hear their reaction when there's something on TV about gays ... 'UGH! It makes me sick!' they say.
>
> (Sue)

But we're not always right

> A good friendship ... that went out of the window ... and then friends who you think wouldn't be supportive have just rallied.
>
> (Joanne)

Sometimes we test reactions first

> I told my mam. It was a no-go area. I sort of tested the ground and said, 'Look, I'm only joking.'
>
> (Anne)

> When I go to college, I'm going to gauge out what other people's opinions are first.
>
> (Lin, who was outed at school)

We all contemplate coming out differently (Alyson 1991). We may give hints, sound out others' attitudes, use our 'instincts' and past experiences, in assessing the risks.

Sometimes we plan coming out

Julie wrote to an agony aunt who gave her a lesbian help-line number.

> I arranged to meet someone in town … It was just really good being with someone I could be honest with.

Before coming out to her family, Joanne

> left home, put myself on the housing list … made sure I was established.

Eleven per cent of lesbian and gay teenagers are thrown out of home when they initially come out to their family (McMillan 1989).

Other situations may be catalysts for coming out; some may be unplanned

> I tend to blurt things out.
>
> (Sue)

> The reason I told my mum was because I was really miserable … she was funny for days … she said, would I think about going to the doctor because of being a lesbian.
>
> (Julie)

Some women feel their life experiences have been so powerful they must come out (Markowe 1996). Both Elsa and Sue were aware they were attracted to women in their teens, had been married for some years and had become disabled afterwards.

> Being told that I had a disabling illness, you suddenly think, 'I've only got one life.'
>
> (Elsa)

Sue felt she could no longer cope with her life as it was and took an overdose. It resulted in permanent loss of balance and total blindness. But

> at least it got me out of what I was in and also led to my first relationship.
>
> (Sue)

If we feel we have no power or choice in our lives, isolation and despair can result (Outright 1991). Given that the accepted proportion of lesbians and gay men is one in ten of the population, the actual suicide rate is often significantly higher (30 per cent of all suicides in the USA are *young* lesbians or gay men, Byrne and Larkin 1994).

Sometimes we are 'outed' and are denied a choice

After being outed at school by heterosexual friends, Lin said,

> The first day, I remember being *so terrified* when I came into school.

> I was outed at work and it wasn't my choice. What right has someone else to do that to me?
>
> (Pauline, who was outed by another lesbian)

As Signorile (1995) says, control over our coming-out process is crucial. It is part of feeling in control of our whole life. Unfortunately, control is not always possible, and is always limited.

Other factors influencing coming out

How important the person or situation is to us

If it is someone new or insignificant:

> I can pretend that I'm straight ... I think it's okay not to tell them. I don't think it's any of their business.
>
> (Asantewaa)

> If I felt I was getting really close to them ... they were talking about their boyfriend, then I'd start to want to.
>
> (Julie)

> I wanted everybody who was important to know about it.
>
> (Trish)

> I don't operate a policy of concealment ... if people want to know they ask me and if I want to tell them I'll tell them ... It's got to be relevant.
>
> (Angela)

Julie, Trish and Ruth all said the women's movement helped facilitate coming out. So, clearly, timing and context are important too.

Sometimes we feel that we 'need' to be out

> Part of it is just a statement: 'There are lesbians about – *don't* assume I'm heterosexual.'
>
> (Tracy)

Anne gathered that she was the first lesbian at a factory where she worked.

> It was like, let them know from the beginning ... if you don't like what you see, just leave it alone.

Also, before she came out, Anne said,

> I had this violent streak, it was like I was denying it ... I used to drink a lot.

> I think you have to for your own sanity ... and talking about it normalizes it as well.
>
> (Asantewaa)

We contemplate *risk*. Is it important enough? What is the possible outcome? As Brosnan (1996: 29) says, 'although coming out is often thought of as being disruptive ... it is generally done in an attempt to get closer'. It is difficult to feel close to others if we cannot be ourselves. Coming out also helps us to meet other lesbians as friends and lovers.

At other times we many consciously avoid coming out for a variety of reasons

Geeta is not out to her family or at work and does not see it as problematic:

> I'm a very private and contained person.

She feels that this is her personality.

We fear rejection and being perceived negatively. Pauline is not out to her family:

My father's very homophobic ... I'm too frightened to find out and I wouldn't want that to isolate me from my mother.

I keep my private life very separate to my work life ... if I was settled and loved my job I might take more of a risk.

(Diane)

You 'de-dyke' the house, taking your books down, your posters down ... it's their problem, but you don't want to offend them.

(Asantewaa)

False stereotypes and assumptions and our decision-taking

As Jones (1988) and Hayfield (1995) highlight, heterosexuals often see lesbians as predatory sexual beings, invalidating our notions of ourselves as whole people.

You suddenly become a sexual being ... you're not Pauline ... it's suddenly Pauline the lesbian.

the danger of people knowing I was gay before they knew *me* ... people do not see past the label, no matter how educated they think they are ... I don't want to be known as the residential dyke.

(Diane)

Angela says that certain heterosexual women

assume you fancy them. I usually say to them, 'Don't flatter yourself!'

Trish felt unsafe about being out in one work environment and avoided personal conversation:

On one level I don't care what they think of me, on another level I wonder if they see me as this frumpy, grey-haired, middle-aged ... do they think I've got no sexuality?

Anne found heterosexuals' questions about her being a lesbian rather predictable.

'What do you actually *do*?' and that's *all* they want to get down to.

Tracy told her family about being abused at the same time as she came out as a lesbian:

People always connect the two – *always*.

Stereotypes have implications for lesbians coming out in certain work environments

Hall Carpenter Archives (1989), Neild and Pearson (1992) show that lesbians who work with children or young people can feel especially stigmatized if they come out.

It's like you are dirty, you're ill, there's something wrong with you and you're going to molest the children all of a sudden.

(Pauline)

The simple act of wanting to comfort an upset young woman can be distorted:

I didn't want them to think, 'Oh, she's a lesbian ... she touched me up.'

(Trish)

The disturbing consequence is that we sometimes internalize homophobia and project on to others what we fear they are thinking:

These are my feelings, aren't they?

(Trish)

Other jobs or situations involving physical contact, e.g. massage, evoke similar fears among lesbians. Yet coming out as a worker can help facilitate other lesbians' coming out.

One of the young women I worked with very closely did come out and that felt really good.

(Tracy)

Clearly, what heterosexuals take for granted is a stressful process for lesbians, influenced by context and our past experiences.

Sexuality is not the only factor influencing how we experience coming out. As Trenchard and Warren (1984) state, there are other pressures that impact on this process. Oppression relating to disability, race, age are all experienced by many lesbians and, as Dominelli (1988) says, they are often experienced not independently but simultaneously.

The impact of other oppressions

Brosnan (1996) and Appleby (1994) suggest that to be lesbian and disabled is to be doubly stigmatized. Disabled women face being de-sexualized, while lesbians face being intensively sexualized, resulting in very distorted and contradictory images.

> If you're an out dyke, you're an abnormal human being, but if you're disabled, you're not human at all.
>
> (Elsa)

Home helps visit Sue every day – because she is blind she has constantly to think about what may be lying around the house that could 'out' her:

> Some of them are just – Shock! Horror! I'm not going in that house again, she might jump on me … I have a drawer where I hide things … unless you can trust them a hundred per cent, it's better to keep it this way because they just don't understand about sexuality.
>
> (Sue)

Because Sue cannot see, she fears being unknowingly 'outed' when she visits gay pubs and clubs, or going to a holiday home for disabled people and not being out there.

> I don't want to risk the chance of losing it.

Sometimes Sue's lesbian friends may slip up and say something in front of others:

> and I'm waiting for a reaction and with not being able to see it's very difficult to pick up.

Another issue that can affect coming out is the inaccessibility of gay venues. Loud music, low lighting, crowds and stairs can all prevent some lesbians with disabilities from accessing the support and social events available to able-bodied lesbians. This can add to stress and isolation.

> There are loads of places you can't go to as disabled lesbians.
>
> (Elsa)

Oppressions are not experienced separately and our priorities may constantly shift depending upon our circumstances at any given time.

> If I'm in an all-white situation then it's going to be race. If I'm in an all-white group and able-bodied, then it's ability. If I'm with black women with disabilities then it might be sexuality.
>
> (Angela)

Angela also says about coming out,

> To me it's a very white, middle-class concept.

In relation to this, Cosis-Brown (1992) and Dixon *et al.* (1989) support the view that coming out may be more immediately relevant and more easily prioritized by white lesbians than for other groups with different priorities. Coming out for black lesbians can have the same positive consequences as for white lesbians: empowerment, a sense of relief and an ability to be oneself (Mason-John and Okorrowa 1995). *Negotiating* coming out, however, can be a far more complex and stressful process than for white able-bodied women. Black lesbians have to cope with the stress of racism. Black mothers face added discrimination. Some lesbians could face deportation if they have been married. For an Iranian lesbian this could result in the death penalty for her sexuality (Mason-John and Okorrowa 1995). There may be a dilemma for a black lesbian anticipating coming out to her family and friends who provide protection from racism. She may lose their vital support in a racist society, perhaps to face racism from within the lesbian community (Suriyaprakasam 1995).

It is clear why coming out can be seen as a white (and often able-bodied middle-class) concept. For lesbians facing other oppressions, there may be more to weigh up, and as a result coming out may not be considered a safe option. 'We have to struggle to find a way of personally negotiating both oppressions' (Cosis-Brown 1992: 209). Parmar (1989) adds that racism can equal the power of homophobia in influencing how and when black lesbians come out.

Kath wondered,

If I was applying for a job, whether this would stop me or interfere with me getting on? It's hard enough being black.

It's funny, I thought I'd met as much prejudice as I was going to meet in my whole life and em, hey! There's more!

(Joanne)

Lin gets angry because

I get enough hassle being Chinese ... why should I get hassle for this?

Being Jewish, Tracy feels that

I really miss out on my culture because I can't be accepted as a dyke.

Bellos (1995) says black women also face being doubly sexualized, as a lesbian by a heterosexist society and as a black woman by a racist society. Black African women may face stereotypes of being 'exotic and uncivilized' and Asian women as being 'exotic and passive' (Hayfield 1995). This could influence decision-making related to coming out. Having taken the risk of coming out, black lesbians could face these same racist stereotypes from white lesbians.

What about the impact of being a lesbian with children?

Brosnan (1996), Rights of Women Lesbian Custody Group (1986) and Dixon *et al.* (1989) all make the point that having children impacts enormously on how lesbians feel about coming out. It can make not only *us* vulnerable but also our children, facing possible harassment, rejection and stigmatization. Lesbians face labels such as 'unfit mothers', often experiencing extreme feelings of powerlessness. This again may be compounded by other oppressions such as racism.

Asantewaa has not come out to her ex-partner because of worries about losing her children:

I think it's to do with my kids and the whole stuff about custody ... people talk about themselves coming out, but I think children do as well.

Romans (1991) highlights the invalidation experienced by lesbian mothers resulting from Section 28 of the Local Government Act 1988. This prevents local authorities from promoting 'homosexuality as a pretended family relationship'. It encourages homophobia and hetero-sexism in a most insidious form, and potentially denies lesbians services of housing authorities, education departments and social services.

Age as a factor in coming out

'Young lesbians ... are, in general, more vulnerable to problems arising from rejection' (Robertson 1995: 8). They can spend an average of up to two years in emotional isolation, unable to tell anyone, says Trenchard (1989). I certainly experienced this and have heard it from others.

As a teenager, Julie started going to a gay disco at a local college, which proved to be a lifeline.

> It ended for the summer and I felt really depressed, I didn't see anyone then all summer.

It is rare for young white lesbians, and rarer for young black lesbians, to find positive role models (Suriyaprakasam 1995). This adds to the isolation experienced by many who can face damaging stereotypes and *no* affirming images.

Older lesbians may face isolation in other forms. Ruth feels she is less bothered about other people's opinions of her now –

> At my age it doesn't make much difference – if they don't accept it, well, that's their hard luck! ... [but] ... the assumptions made about age are dreadful.

Seneviratne (1995) points out that older black lesbians may be more self-confident, but can face isolation as they encounter invisibility and a sense of being the 'only one'. Negotiating coming out in this context could be a painful experience.

Geeta highlights this, when she states that there are very few meeting places for older lesbians, but for younger lesbians 'there are a lot more places to go'.

Support gained from meeting with other lesbians and the sense of community offered by gay venues may be denied older lesbians who are not part of the 'scene'. It could be difficult, therefore, for an older lesbian first thinking of coming out, faced with a minimum of support structures. Also, older women may have had more pressures put on them to lead 'traditional' lives and to marry when they were younger. For lesbians aware of their sexuality from an early age, coming out may never have been an option.

> The sort of background that I came from ... you grew up, got married, that's what you did and that's what I did.
>
> (Elsa)

> A group of friends that ... were all kind of boy-mad ... and I thought that's what I'm supposed to do, and yet just felt absolutely terrible.
>
> (Sue)

When Anne did finally come out

> It was like – yes! like being locked up ... and then finally the door's open and saying, 'You're free now' ... it was brilliant!

As Neild and Pearson (1992) point out, age and disability may interact. Some 'out' older lesbians who have also become disabled may find themselves fearful of losing support or facing the homophobia of carers, and have gone 'back in the closet'. This illustrates that coming out is not a 'once and for all' lifetime event. Age and infirmity may force silence on some lesbians.

The implications for social work

Being homophobic is not simply about the words used, such as calling someone 'queer' or 'dyke'. Homophobia and heterosexism go deeper than the use of language, to assumptions made, what *is not* said or asked of gay people as much as what is, and whether lesbians and gay men feel included and affirmed or isolated. Lesbians do not always have positive views of social work.

Geeta worked in a social work office once:

> Social workers are supposed to be fairly ... sympathetic and feel empathy with their clients ... sometimes they don't ... I thought about it [coming out] but I dropped the idea.

When Pauline was outed at work she said:

Two homophobic staff members were worse after, and one qualified male social worker said, 'But *you're* not like the rest.'

Sue's experience with a male social worker was positive but:

I knew for a fact that he was homosexual.

Since some lesbians choose social work as a career (Hillin 1985), lesbians make up at least 10 per cent of clients, many of whom are homeless teenagers; one in five young lesbians and gay men attempt suicide before the age of 20 (McMillan 1989); and lesbians sometimes find themselves involved in custody cases, it is of concern that sexuality is still a low priority on the social work curriculum, and indeed is often entirely invisible. As Cosis-Brown (1992) states, lesbians still face discrimination in society and within many social work practices, yet the topic is undervalued in the teaching of anti-discrimination. As a result, students, tutors and practitioners often choose not to risk coming out. 'This arises from rational fears of colleagues', employers' and clients' responses' (Cosis-Brown 1992: 209). What is emancipatory action for one lesbian or gay man could mean the 'outing' of another. In voicing our needs we make ourselves *visible* and vulnerable to stigma and labelling, as well as to the positive consequences of openness and honesty. This highlights the contradictory position we often find ourselves in.

Sone (1993) describes the 'lip service' paid to anti-discrimination within social work. Sexuality is seen as embarrassing and stigmatizing, homophobia and heterosexism are still challenged far less than some other forms of discrimination. Does social work hide its homophobia under a veneer of anti-discrimination?

Romans (1991: 14) shows that social workers can sexualize lesbian clients. One lesbian mother was asked 'how many partners I had'. Social workers may focus on sexuality and ignore the client as a whole person *or* ignore the needs of their lesbian client(s) entirely. Social workers need to be aware that Britain has more laws which discriminate against lesbians and gay men than *any other* European country. There is no law which protects them, recognizes their relationships or their partners regarding inheritance, tenancy rights or visiting rights in hospital (Tatchell 1990).

How then can social work begin to deal with homophobia and heterosexism? Social workers themselves can look at their own practice and how they relate to colleagues and clients. Social work courses can begin to properly address sexuality by looking at the range of questions affecting lesbians and gay men. What assumptions are made about people's sexuality? What questions are asked and not asked, when assessing clients or talking to colleagues? What is coming out and what affects it? Hanscombe and Forster (1982) state: 'as far as the law and institutions are concerned, lesbians do not exist. On an official form, for example, there is a space for sex and another for marital status'. These assumptions need to be challenged and such questions replaced by: 'Do you have a partner? How would you describe your sexuality? What are your needs, if any, in relation to your sexuality?' For Sue, whom I interviewed, a home care service employing lesbians and gay men, or which challenged homophobia among its employees, would make her life far less stressful.

McMillan (1989: 31) says that social workers should be aware of the diversity of sexuality at the point of assessment. With the right approach, social workers can enable clients to feel comfortable, accepted and therefore able to come out (if they so wish) by 'enquiring of all clients how they identify their sexuality ... giving them an opportunity to present as a whole person'. Trust and openness could be facilitated *and* appropriate service provision accessed. Social workers need to be aware that lesbians and gay men may feel anxious and suspicious (for good reasons) and may be reticent to talk openly about themselves. Others may choose not to come out because it simply does not feel relevant to them. The issue is about framing questions and practice in a way that is inclusive and not exclusive and heterosexist, a process which facilitates openness if it is deemed relevant *by the client*. Addressing issues related to sexuality, facilitating coming out (if appropriate), could all be initiated and supported by sensitive social work training. This has implications for provision of services as well as creating a safer environment for students, social workers and social work teachers.

Radical changes need to be made within social work. It is not enough to state, 'I am non-judgmental', 'I am not homophobic.' Supporting coming out as a valid option requires challenging homophobic and heterosexist assumptions that are ingrained within institutional practices and belief systems in college, social work departments and individual social workers.

Lesbian and gay sexuality is complex because we can remain hidden (with negative consequences) unless we give ourselves permission to speak out. For many this is a rational decision-making process based on assessment of the level of safety. This is an important point. Lest it be assumed that the experience of being a lesbian is entirely disempowering, it needs to be said that 'empowerment' may not always be about 'giving a voice'. Lesbians exercise power by sometimes choosing not to voice who we are. The emancipatory struggle must exist within this context – that, for lesbians, having a voice is a multi-dimensional choice. We may choose to be visible and speak out at times and remain silent at others. Each decision is part of a fight for freedom and equality, and was true of all the women I interviewed – we are some-times 'out' and sometimes 'in', according to our perception of each situation. Social workers and other professionals need to recognize this, and resist bringing inappropriate pressure to 'speak'.

Conclusion

It will be clear that the contemplation and negotiation of coming out is a complex decision-making process. It is often based on a logical assessment of perceived risk and outcomes. It can affect every area of our lives and is also ongoing and fluid in nature. While coming out is frequently an important issue for lesbians, 'It is often easier for white, middle class, able-bodied women with no children to be open about being lesbian. Those who face other discrimination take more risks by coming out' (Trenchard 1989: 19).

This does not diminish the impact of homophobia and hetero-sexism, but it highlights that oppressions interrelate. It also illustrates that any study of lesbians and coming out would be distorted without taking account of this diversity.

There are many factors which influence our approach to coming out, not least the attitudes and practices of friends, family, work colleagues and the professionals with whom we may come into contact. We may be out or feel forced out by circumstances, but we can exercise some choice and control. In choosing to come out, even if only selectively, we can finally be ourselves – experiencing greater confidence and self-esteem. We can also access support and contact from other lesbians. If we feel unable to come out, we often feel disem-powered and undermined. Many of our interactions are then dominated by a sense of being closeted.

There are occasions when lesbians choose not to be out. A conscious assessment is made of safety and risk given our individual circumstances. This may be particularly true for women facing further prejudice and oppression, such as lesbians with children. We may exer-cise some power and control and *choose* to protect ourselves and others. Thus we minimize our sense of being a victim in the face of oppression. Not coming out, therefore, is not necessarily a negative choice but rather can be a *rational* choice.

I hope I have adequately illustrated why I find the concept of 'lesbians shoving their sexuality down the throats of heterosexuals' offensive and inaccurate. Often a tentative mention of one's sexuality can bring such an attack. In any case, we are merely asking for recognition and are speaking out against prejudice and oppression. As Signorile (1995) points out, lesbians are all 'in' and 'out' of the closet to varying degrees at different points in their lives. Few are ever completely out. It is *vital* that we are allowed to negotiate coming out with as much power and control as possible.

Heterosexuals have their sexuality affirmed constantly because their behaviour is accepted and is therefore the norm. It is because sexuality is socially constructed within a heterosexist context that what heterosexuals take for granted every day of their lives is labelled 'coming out' for lesbians. And then again, 'coming out' does not lead to 'liberation', but to a different kind of oppression. The empowerment entailed in it is as an act of resistance.

References

Appleby, Y. (1994) 'Out in the margins', *Disability and Society* 9(1), 19–32.

Bellos, L. (1995) 'A vision back and forth', in J.V. Mason (ed.), *Talking Black: Lesbians of African and Asian Descent Speak Out*, London and New York: Cassell, 52–71.

Brosnan, J. (1996) *Lesbians Talk – Detonating the Nuclear Family*, London: Scarlet Press.

Byrne, S. and Larkin, J. (1994) *Coming Out – A Book for Lesbians and Gay Men of All Ages*, New York: Martello Books.

Carabine, J. (1996) 'Empowering sexualities', in B. Humphries (ed.), *Critical Perspectives on Empowerment*, Birmingham: Venture Press, 17–34.

Card, C. (1995) *Lesbian Choices*, New York: Columbia University Press

Cosis-Brown, H. (1992) 'Lesbians, the state and social work practice', in M. Langan and L. Day (eds), *Women, Oppression and Social Work*, London: Routledge, 201–19.

——(1998) *Social Work and Sexuality: Working with Lesbians and Gay Men*, London: Macmillan Press.

Dixon, J., Salvat, G. and Skeats, J. (1989) 'North London Young Lesbian Group: Specialist Work within the Youth Service', in C. Jones and P. Mahony (eds), *Learning Our Lines: Sexuality and Social Control in Education*, London: The Women's Press, 232–48.

Dominelli, L. (1988) *Anti-Racist Social Work*, London: Macmillan Education.

Epstein, D. and Johnson, R. (1994) 'On the straight and narrow: the heterosexual presumption, homophobia and schools', in D. Epstein (ed.), *Challenging Lesbian and Gay Inequalities in Education*, Buckingham: Open University Press, 179–230.

234   *Helen Williamson*

Graham, H. (1993) *Hardship and Health in Women's Lives*, New York, London: Harvester Wheatsheaf.

Hall, M. (1993) 'Private experiences in the public domain: lesbians in organisations', in J. Hearn, D.L. Sheppard, P. Tancred-Sheriff and G. Burrell (eds), *The Sexuality of Organisations*, London: Sage, 125–38.

Hall Carpenter Archives (1989) *Inventing Ourselves – Lesbian Life Stories*, London: Routledge.

Hanscombe, G.E. and Forster, J. (1982) *Rocking the Cradle: Lesbian Mothers, A Challenge in Family Living*, Glasgow: Sheba Feminist Publishers.

Hayfield, A. (1995) 'Several faces of discrimination', in V. Mason-John (ed.), *Talking Black: Lesbians of African and Asian Descent Speak Out*, London: Cassell, 186–206.

Hicks, S. and McDermott, J. (eds) (1999) *Lesbian and Gay Fostering and Adoption*, London: Jessica Kingsley.

Hillin, A. (1985) 'When You Stop Hiding Your Sexuality', *Social Work Today*, 19 (4 November), 18–19.

Jones, R. (1988) 'With respect to lesbians', *Nursing Times*, 18 May, 84(20), 48–9.

Kitzinger, C. (1987) *The Social Construction of Lesbianism*, London: Sage.

Lorde, A. (1985) *I Am Your Sister: Black Women Organising Across Sexualities*, New Jersey: Women of Color Press.

Lovell, A. (1995) *When Your Child Comes Out*, London: Sheldon Press.

McMillan, S. (1989) 'Lesbians and gay men need services too', *Social Work Today*, 6 July, 20(43), 31.

Markowe, L.A. (1996) *Re-defining the Self – Coming Out As A Lesbian*, Cambridge: Polity Press.

Marland Hitchcock, J. and Skodal Wilson, H. (1992) 'Personal risking: lesbian self-disclosure of sexual orientation to professional health care providers', *Nursing Research*, May/June, 41(3), 178–83.

Mason-John, V. and Okorrowa, A. (1995) 'A minefield in the garden: black lesbian sexuality', in V. Mason-John (ed.), *Talking Black: Lesbians of African and Asian Descent Speak Out*, London: Cassell, 72–93.

Mohanty, C.T. (1991) 'Under Western eyes: feminist scholarship and colonial discourses', in C.T. Mohanty, A. Russo and L. Torres (eds), *Third World Women and the Politics of Feminism*, Indianapolis: Indiana University Press, 51–80.

Neild, S. and Pearson, R. (1992) *Women Like Us*, London: The Women's Press.

Outright (1991) *I Think I Might Be A Lesbian ... Now What Do I Do?*, London: Lesbian Information Service.

Parmar, P. (1989) 'Black lesbians', in Boston Women's Health Book Collective, *The New Our Bodies Ourselves*, Harmondsworth: Penguin, 221–6.

Rakusen, J. (1989) 'Relationships: some issues for us all', in Boston Women's Health Book Collective, *The New Bodies Ourselves*, Harmondsworth: Penguin, 191–202.

Rich, A. (1980) 'Introduction', in J.P. Stanley and S.J. Wolfe *Coming Out Stories*, Watertown, Mass.: Persephone Press, xi–xiii.

Rights of Women Lesbian Custody Group (1986) *Lesbian Mother's Legal Handbook*, London: The Women's Press.

Robertson, R. (1995) *Lesbian or Gay – Telling Your Parents*, London: FFLAG (Families and Friends of Lesbians and Gays).

Romans, P. (1991) 'Women with much to offer', *Community Care*, 14 March, 14–15.

Seneviratne, S. (1995) '… and some of us are older', in V. Mason-John (ed.), *Talking Black: Lesbians of African and Asian Descent Speak Out*, London: Cassell, 108–29.

Signorile, M. (1995) *Outing Yourself: How to Come Out as Lesbian or Gay to Your Family, Friends and Colleagues*, London: Abacus.

Sone, K. (1993) 'Coming out at work', *Community Care*, 7 October, 18.

Suriyaprakasam, S. (1995) 'Some of us are younger', in V. Mason-John (ed.), *Talking Black: Lesbians of African and Asian Descent Speak Out*, London: Cassell, 94–107.

Tatchell, P. (1990) *Out in Europe: A Guide to Lesbian and Gay Rights in Thirty European Countries*, London: Channel Four Television Publications.

Trenchard, L. (1989) *Being Lesbian*, London: GMP Publishers.

Trenchard, L. and Warren, H. (1984) *Something To Tell You*, London: London Gay Teenage Group.

Truman, C. (1994) 'Feminist challenges to traditional research: have they gone far enough?', in B. Humphries and C. Truman (eds), *Re-thinking Social Research*, Aldershot: Avebury, 21–36.

Weeks, J. (1990) *Coming Out*, London: Quartet Books.

——(1987) 'Questions of identity', in P. Caplan (ed.), *The Cultural Construction of Sexuality*, London: Routledge, 31–51.

Williamson, H. (1997) 'In or out? How lesbians negotiate and experience coming out', unpublished MA dissertation, Manchester Metropolitan University.

Yeatman, A. (1993) 'Voice and representation in the politics of difference', in S. Gunew and A. Yeatman, *Feminism and the Politics of Difference*, London: Allen and Unwin, 228–45.

Index